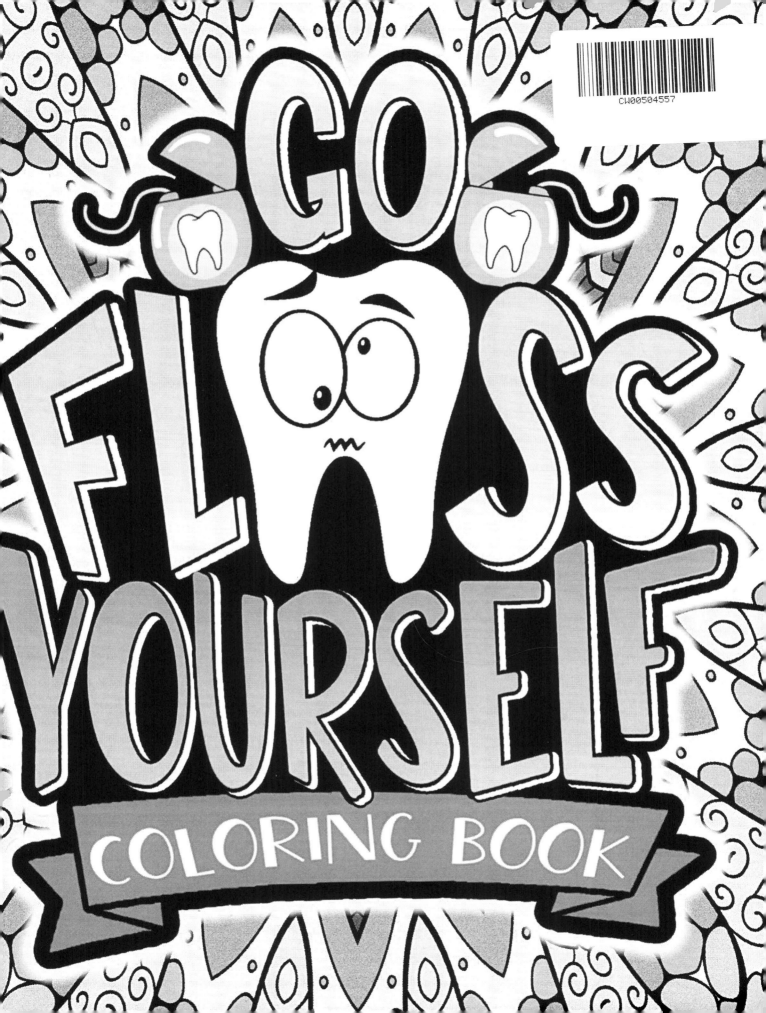

GO
FLOSS
YOURSELF
COLORING BOOK

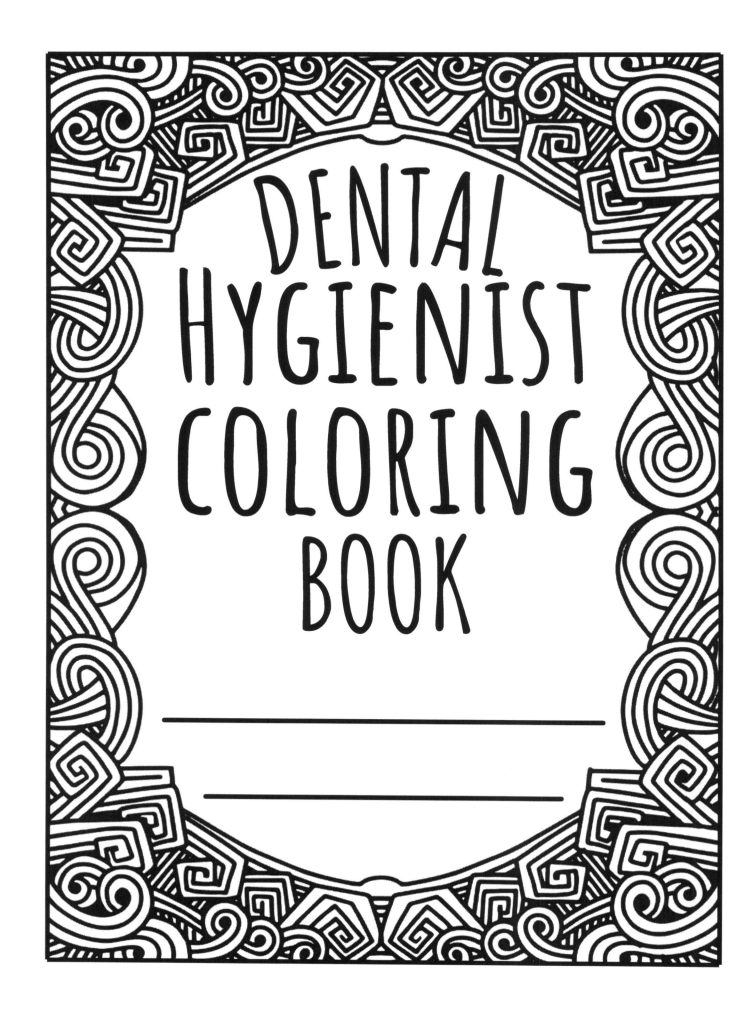

# DENTAL HYGIENIST COLORING BOOK

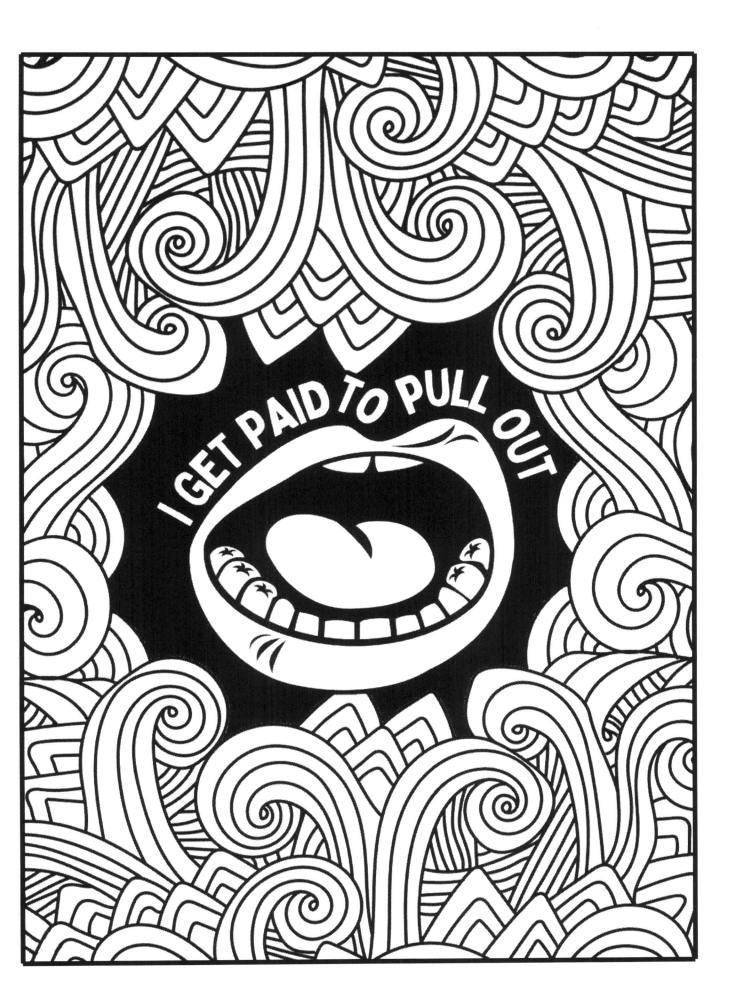

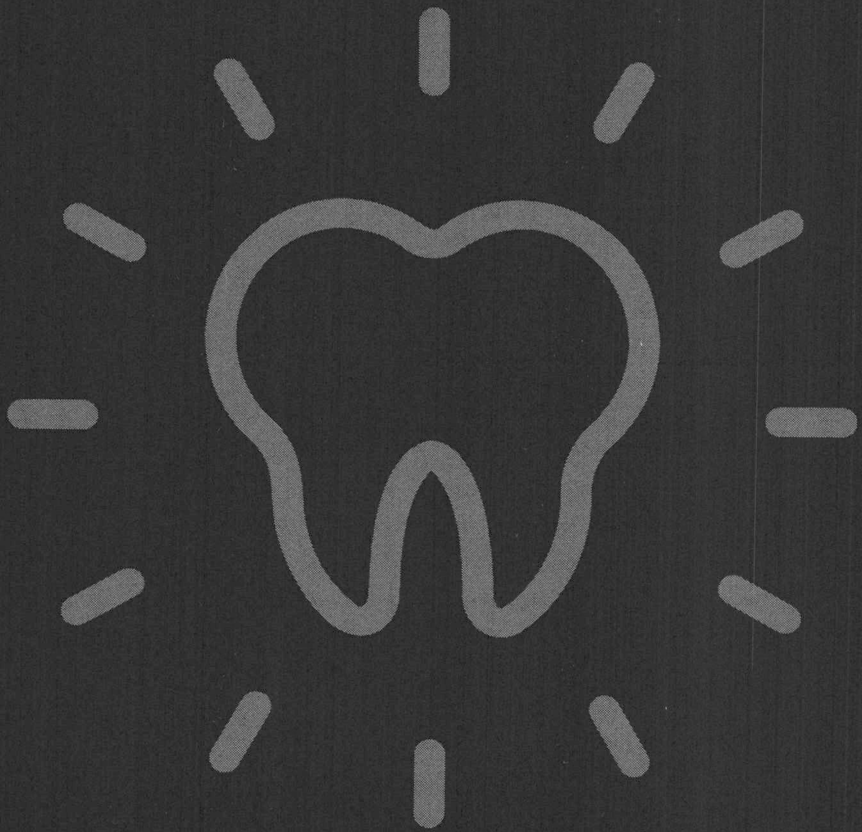

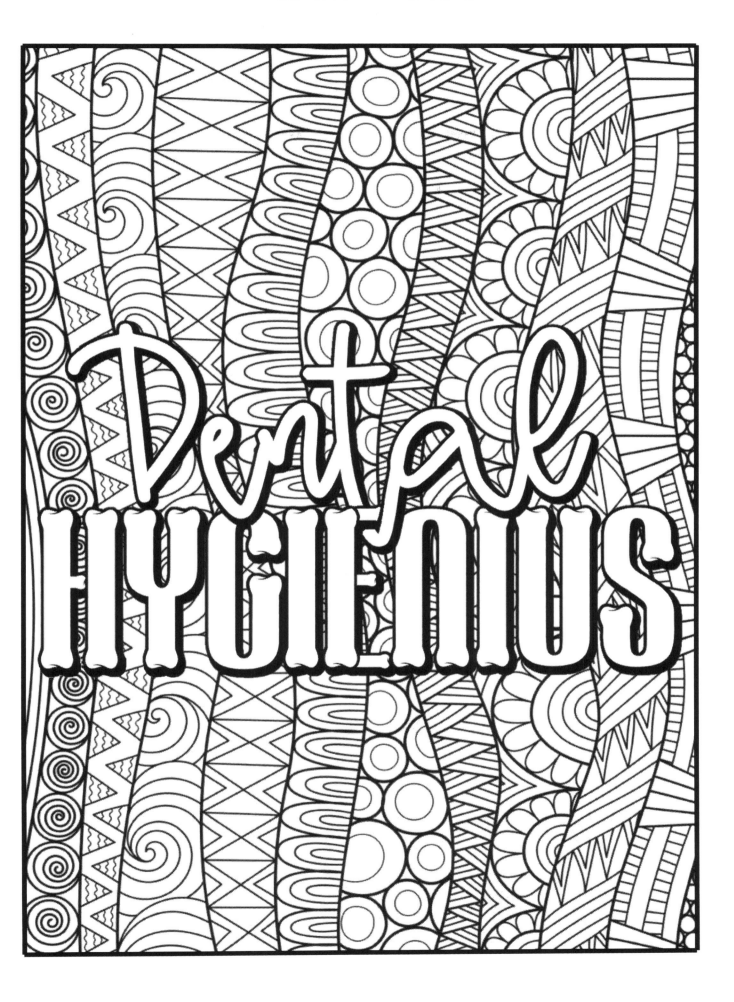

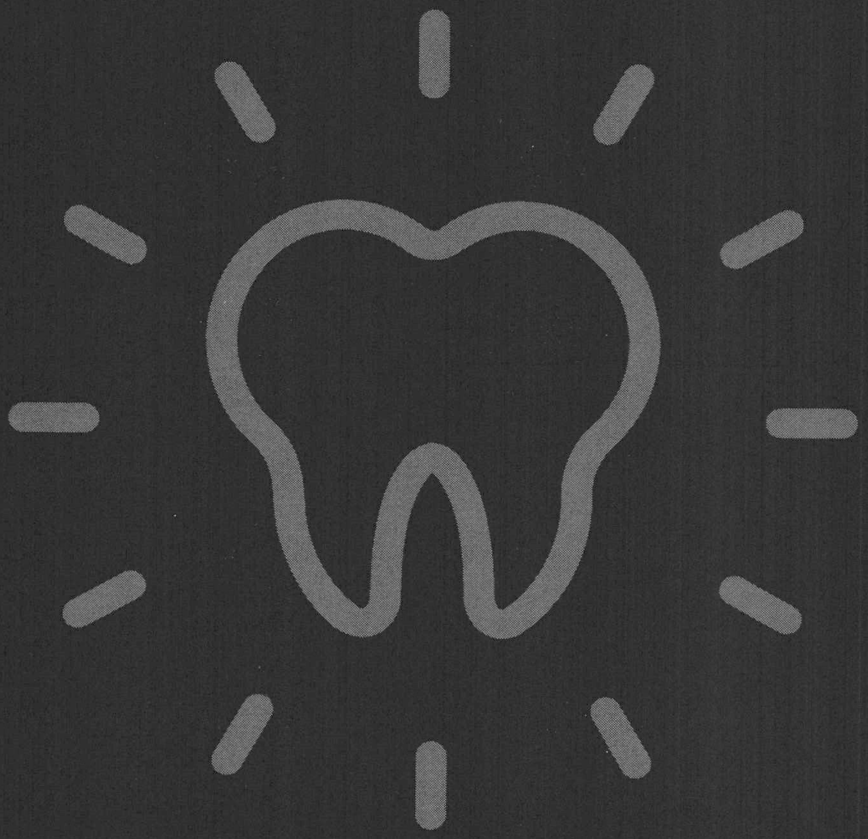

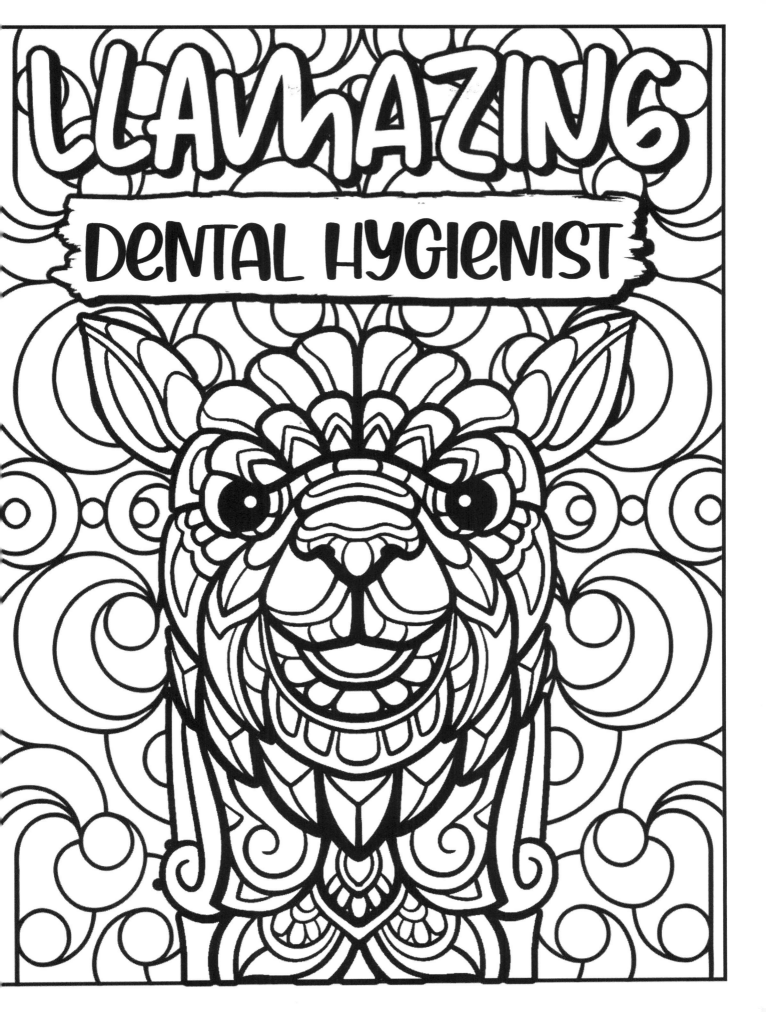

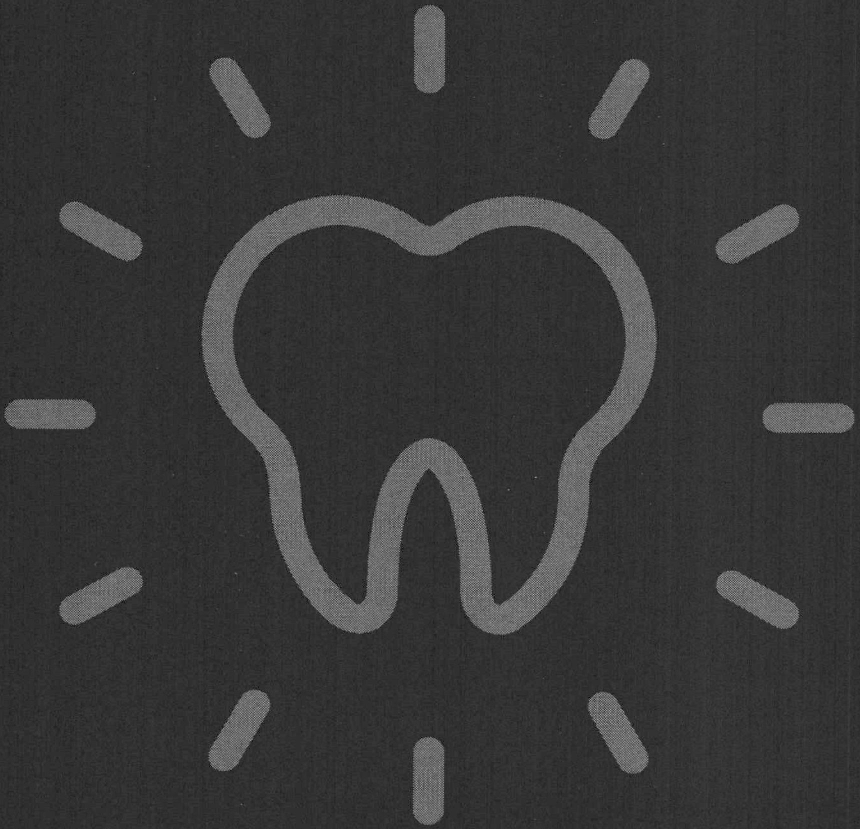

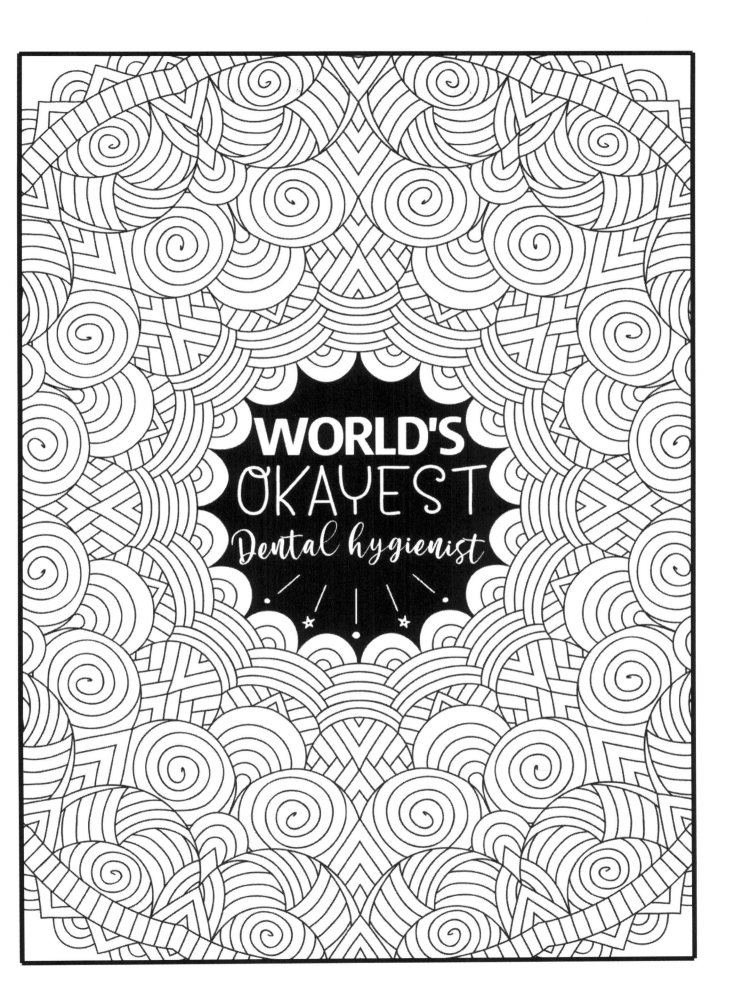

WORLD'S OKAYEST Dental hygienist

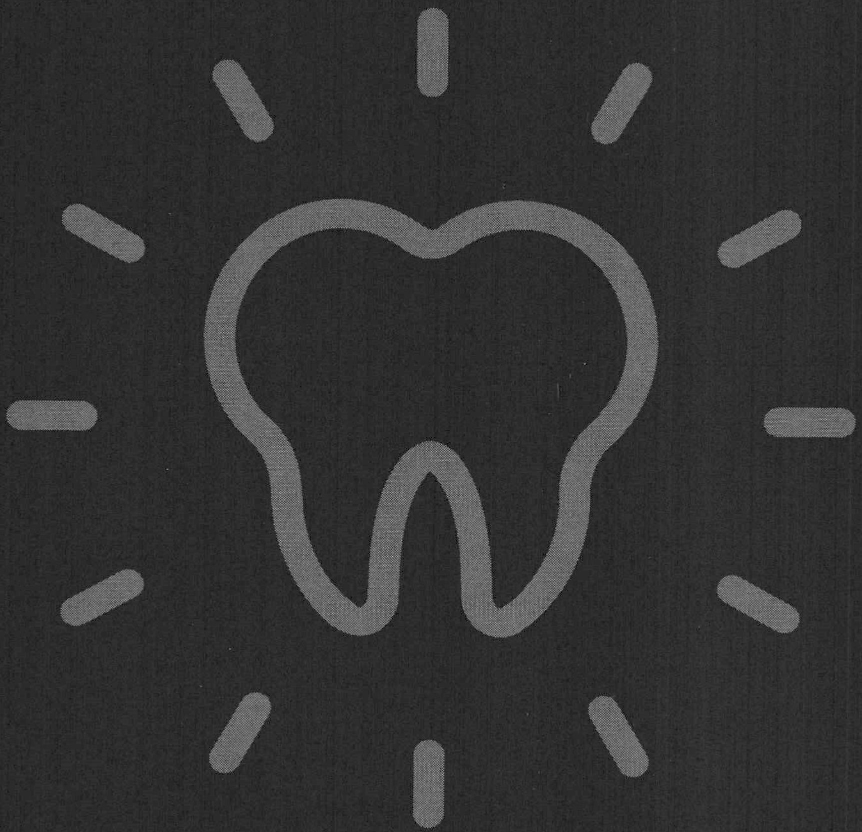

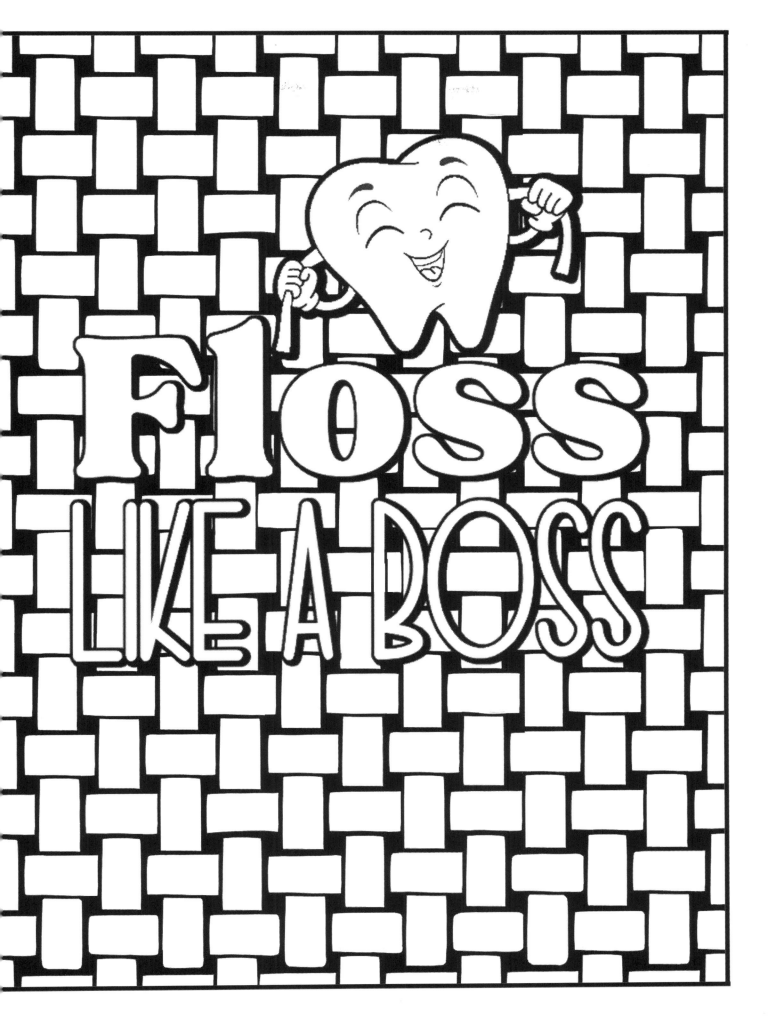

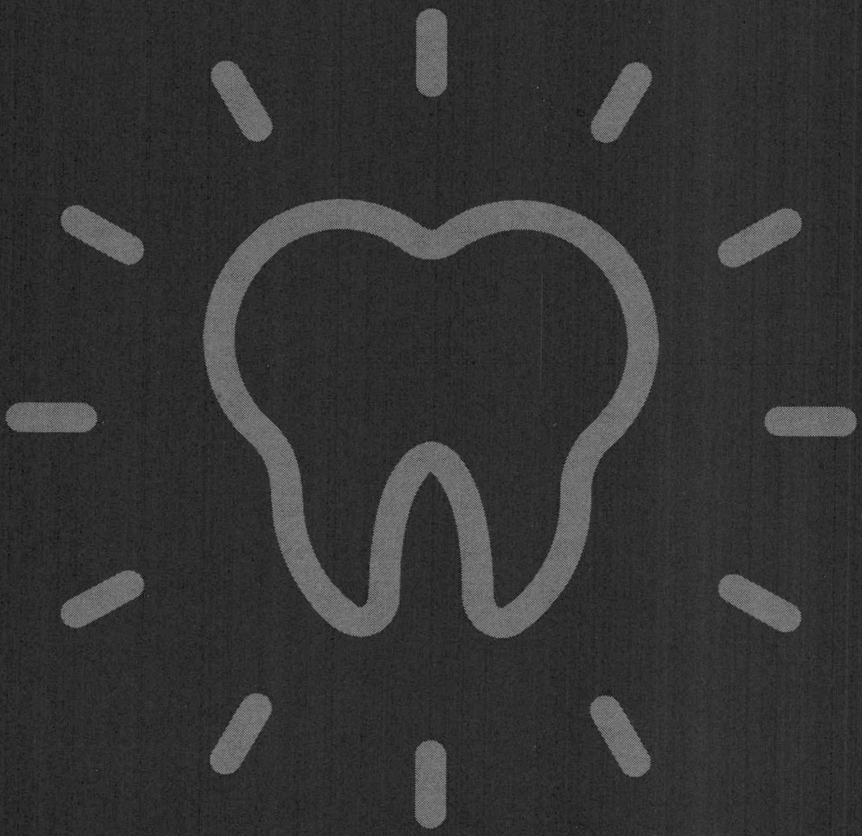

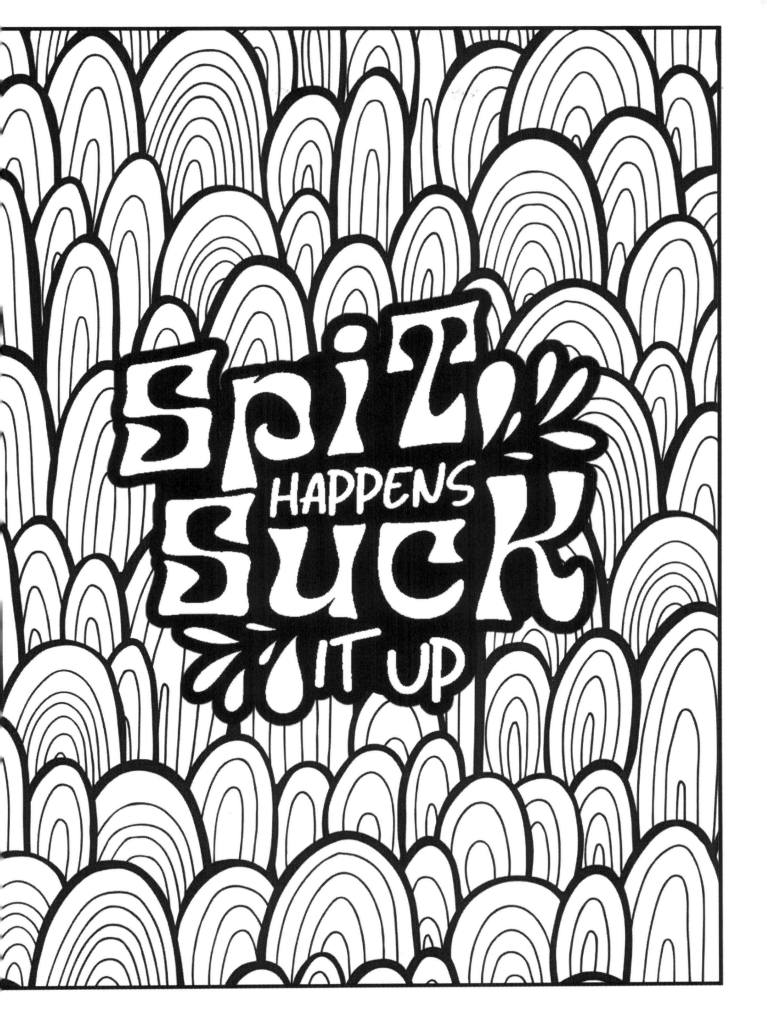

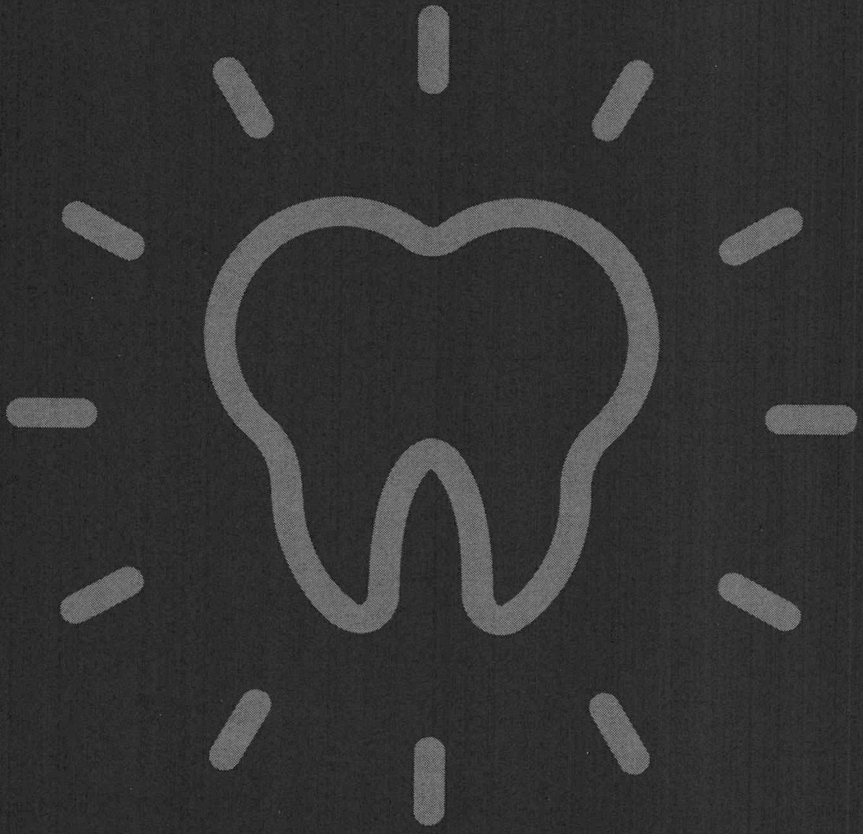

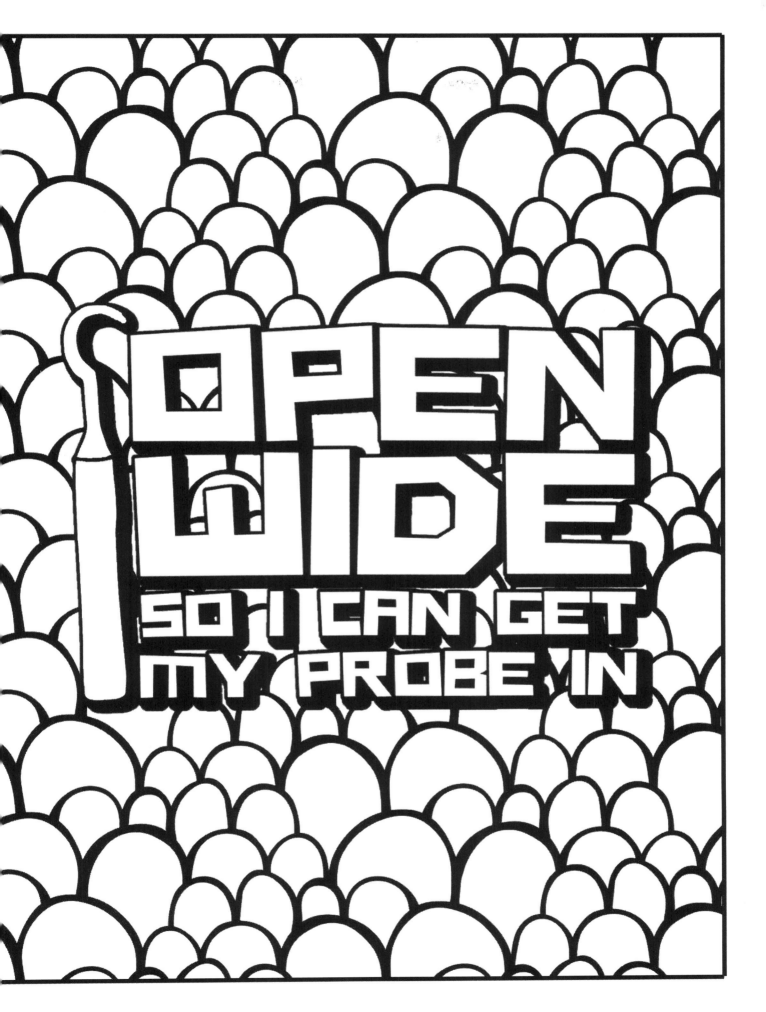

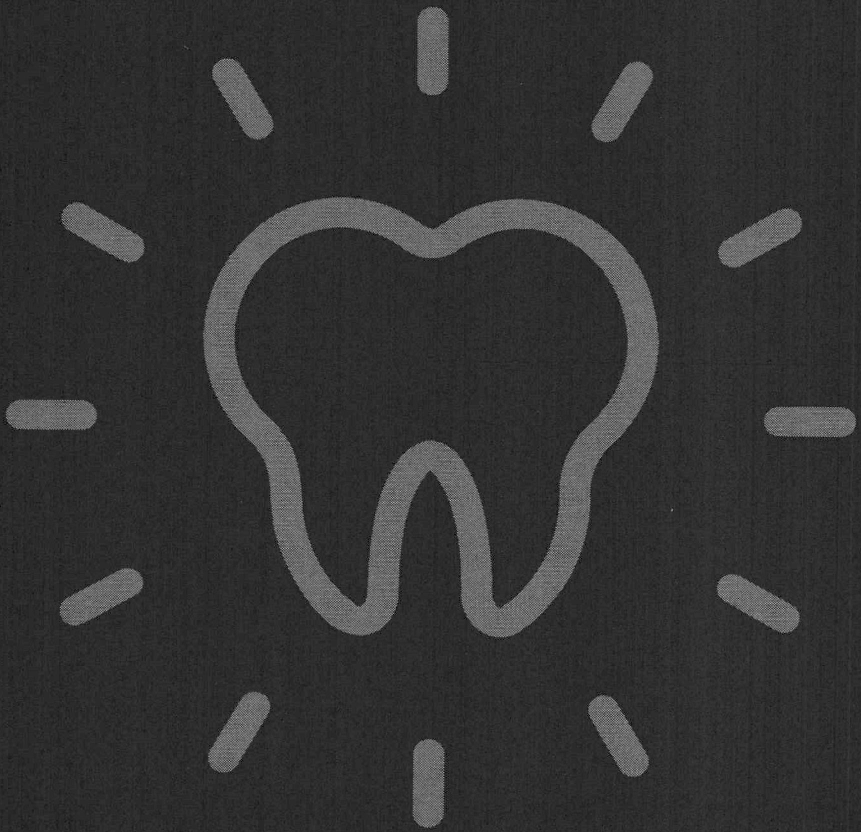

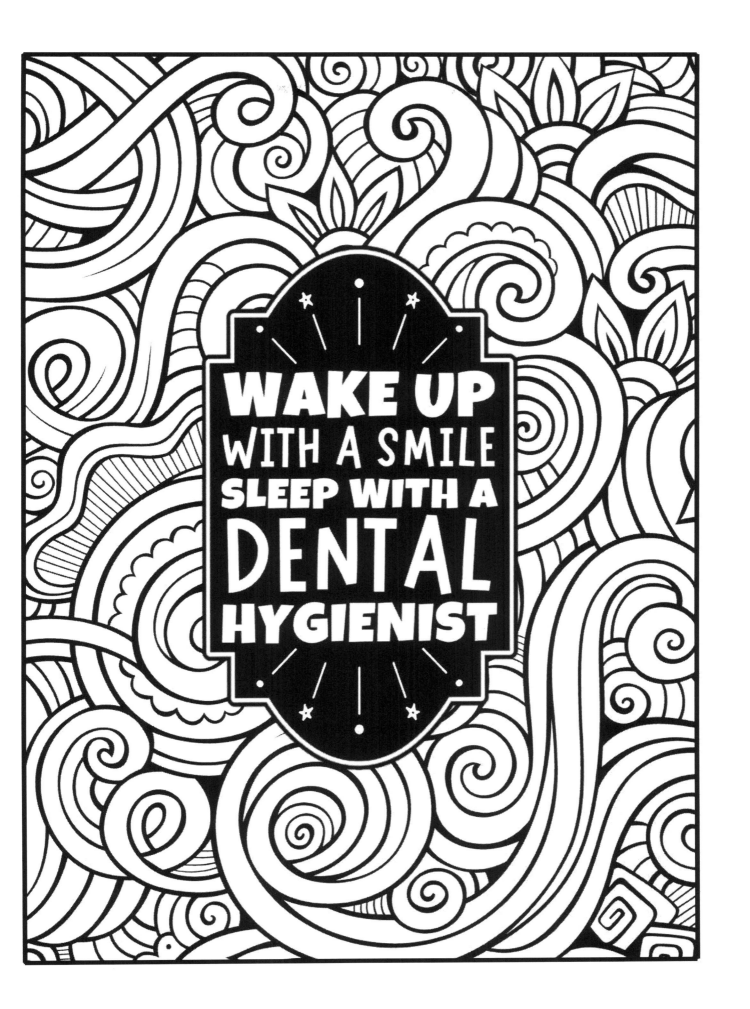

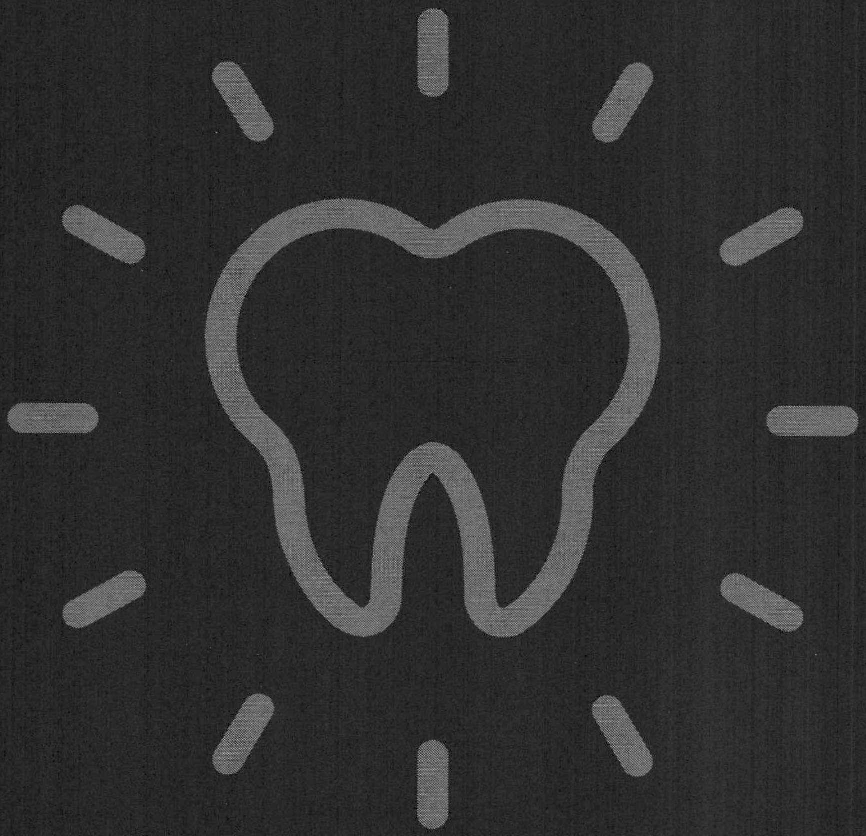

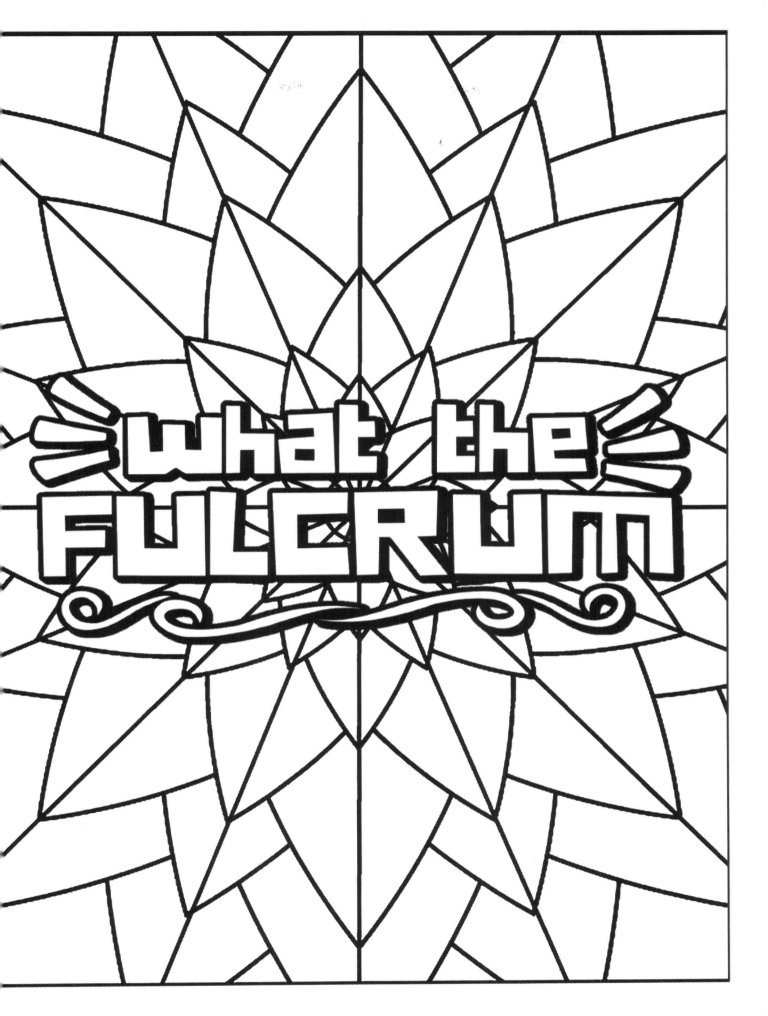

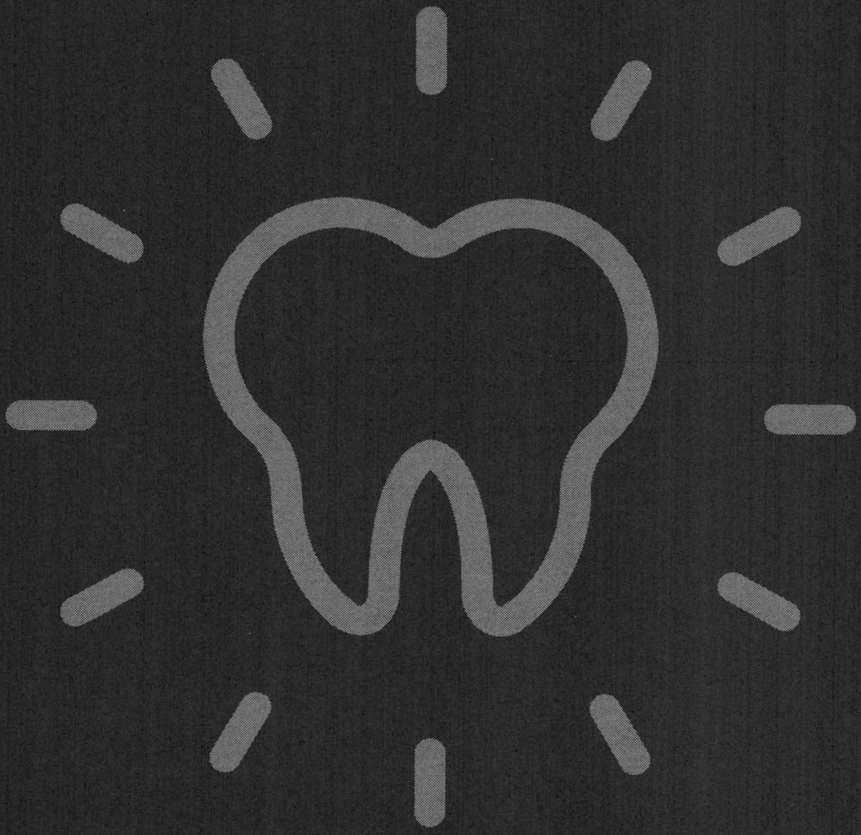

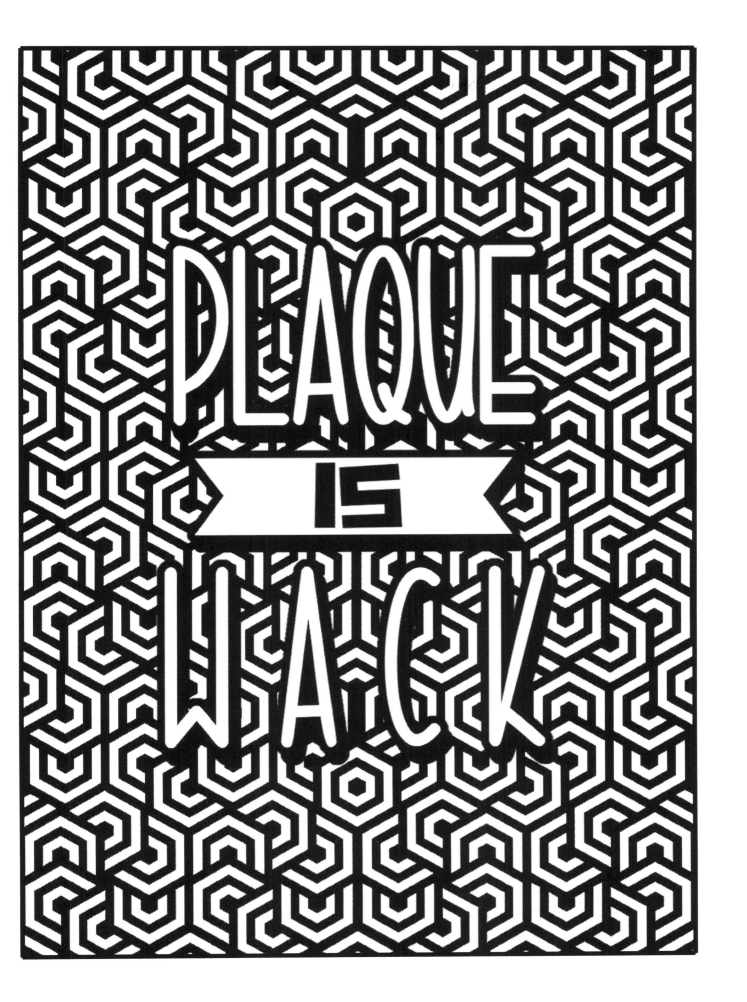

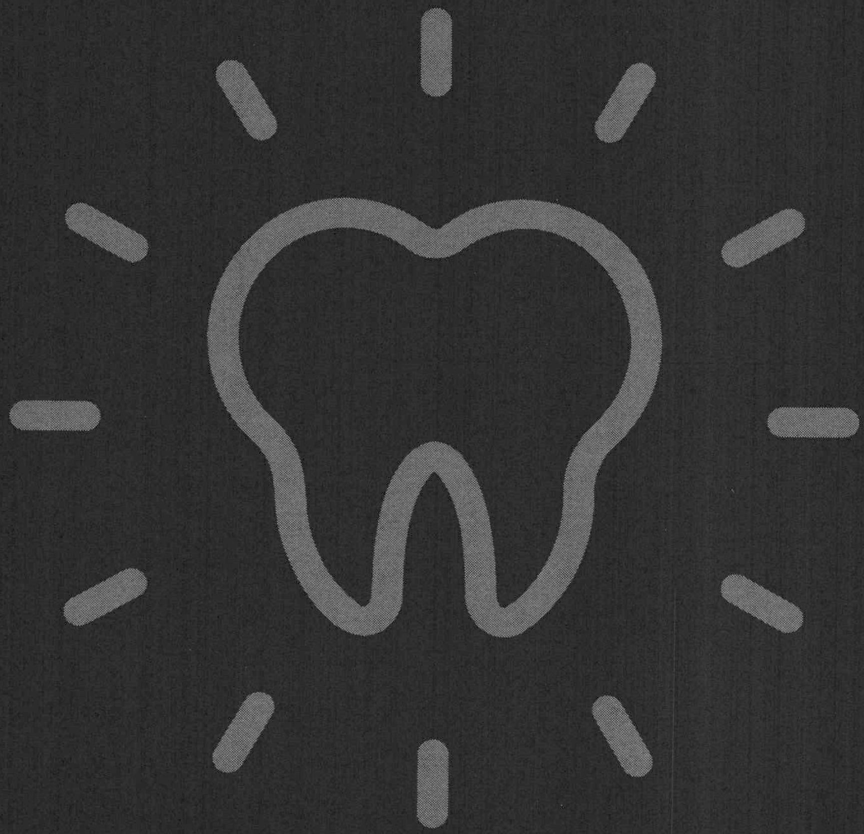

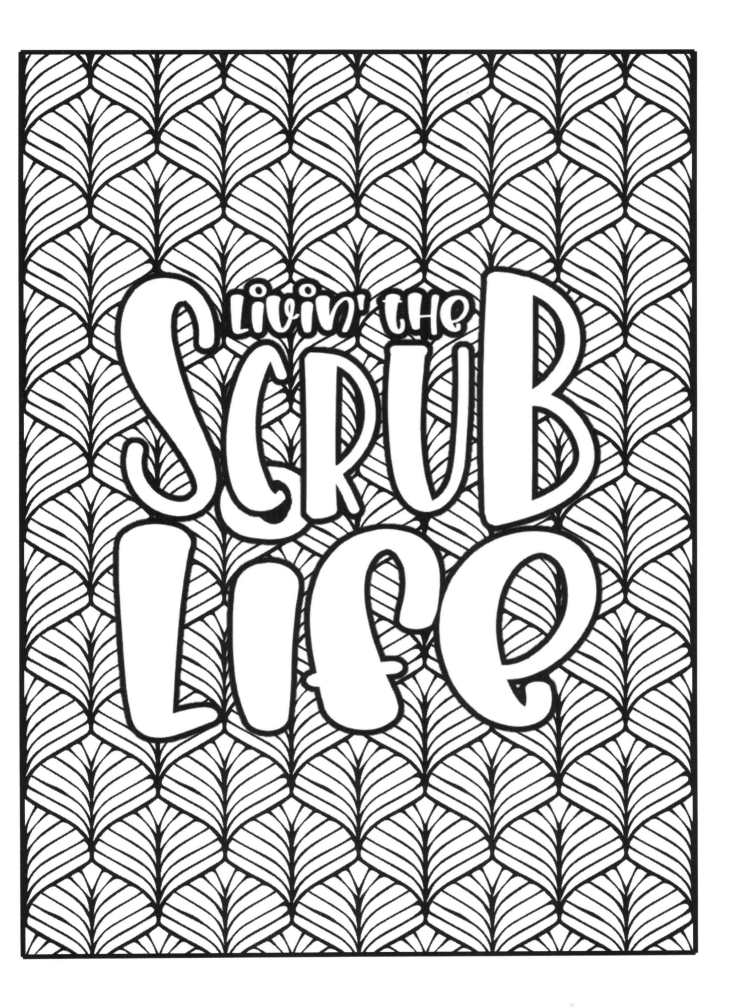

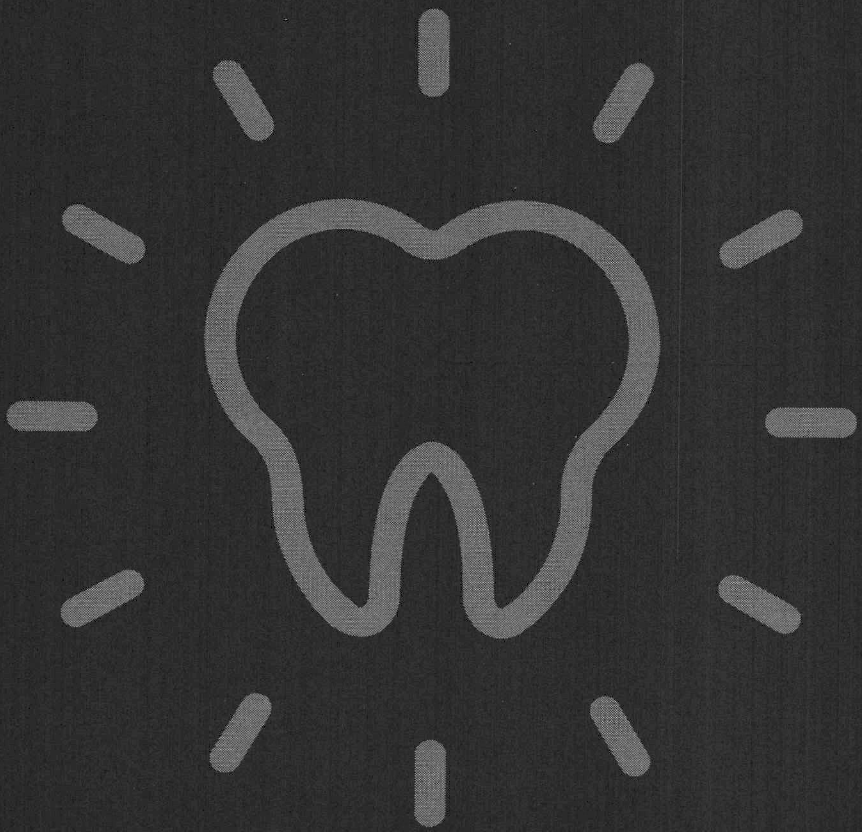

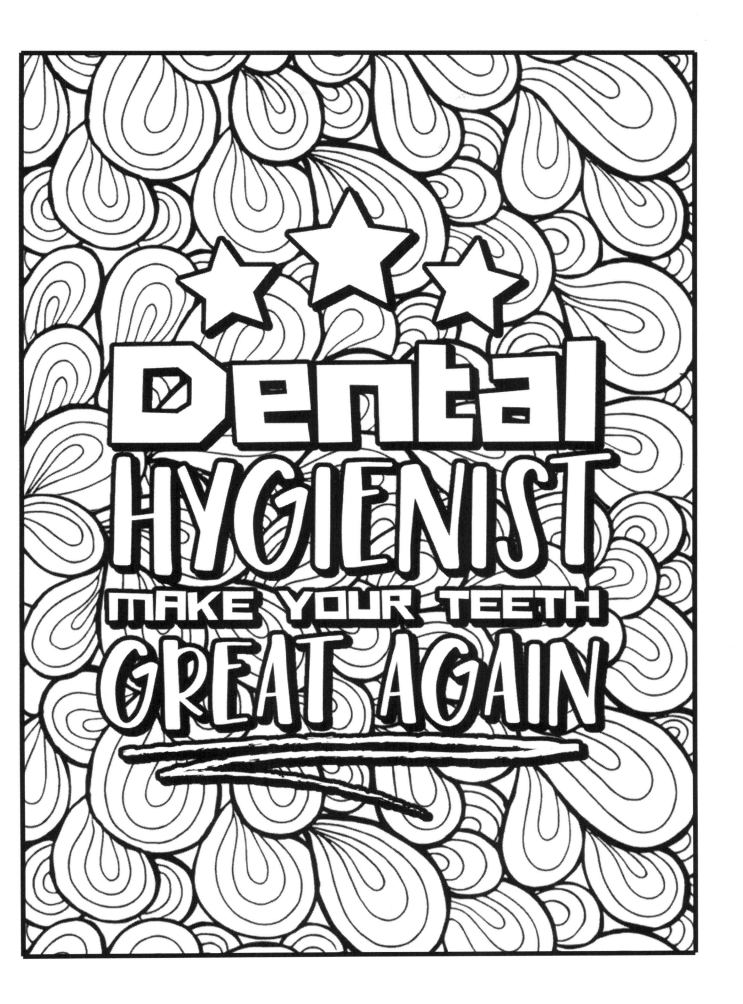

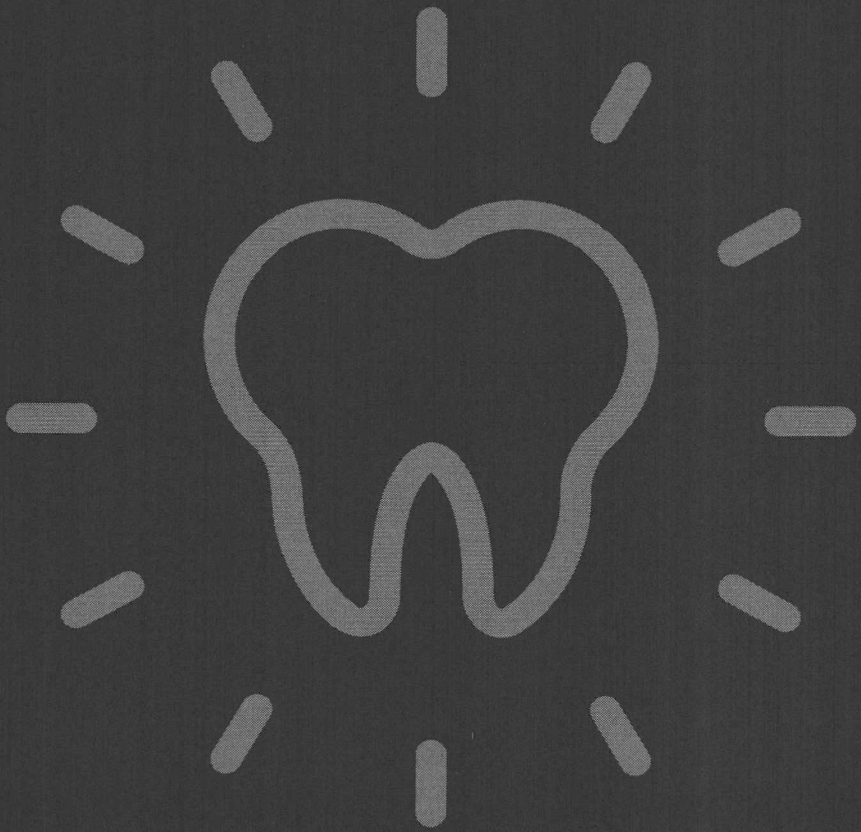

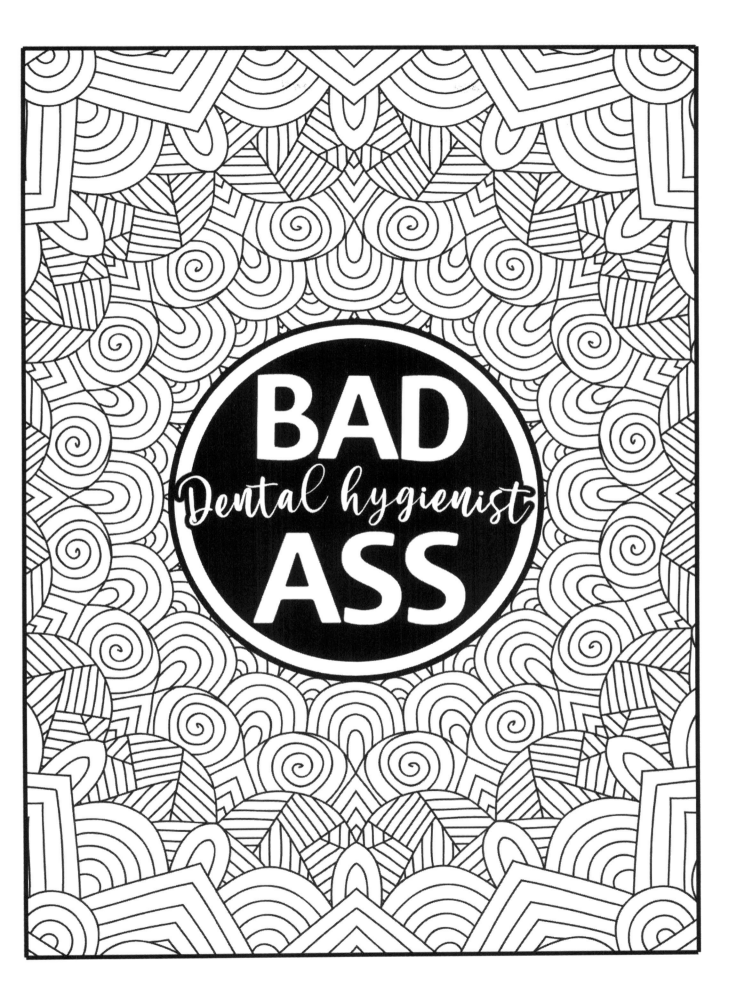

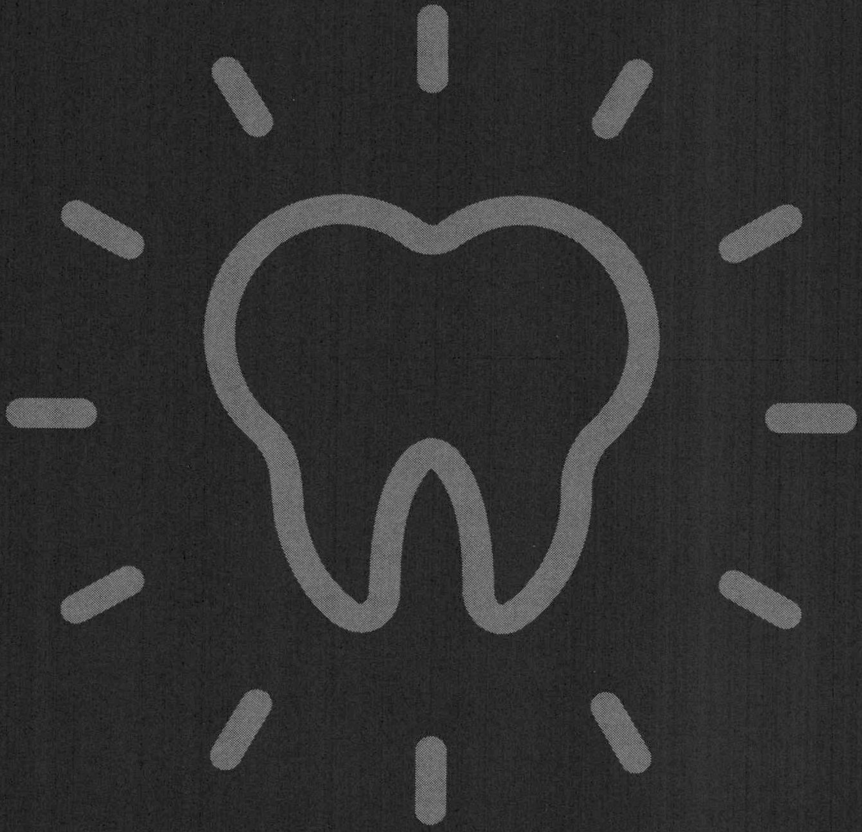

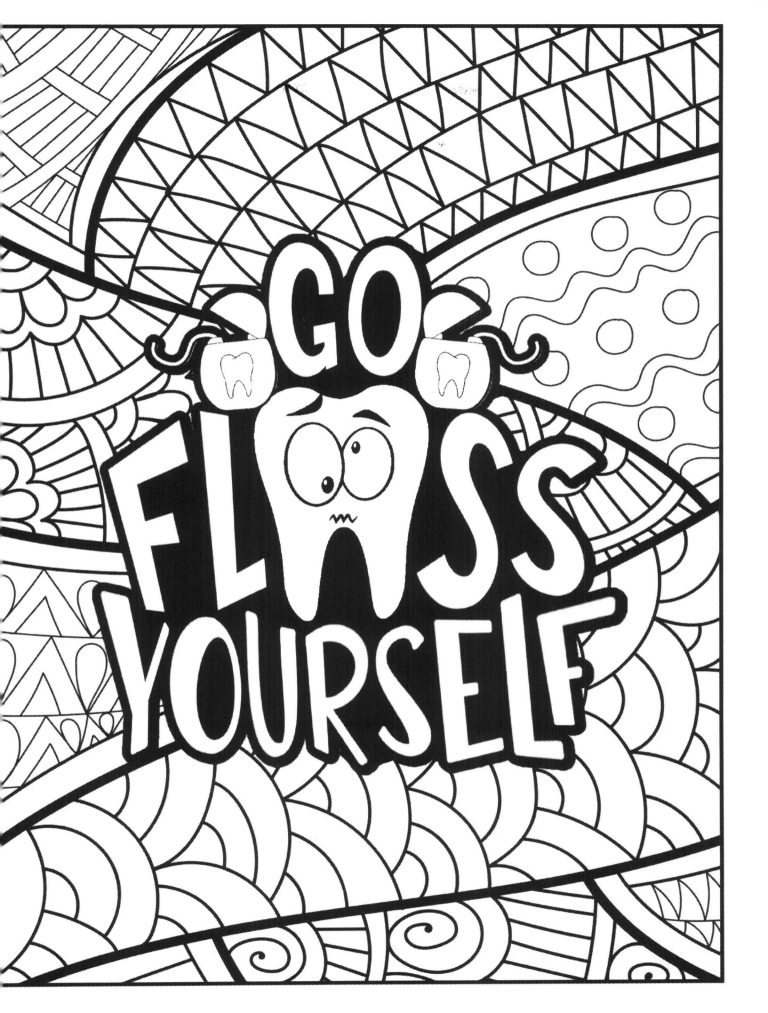

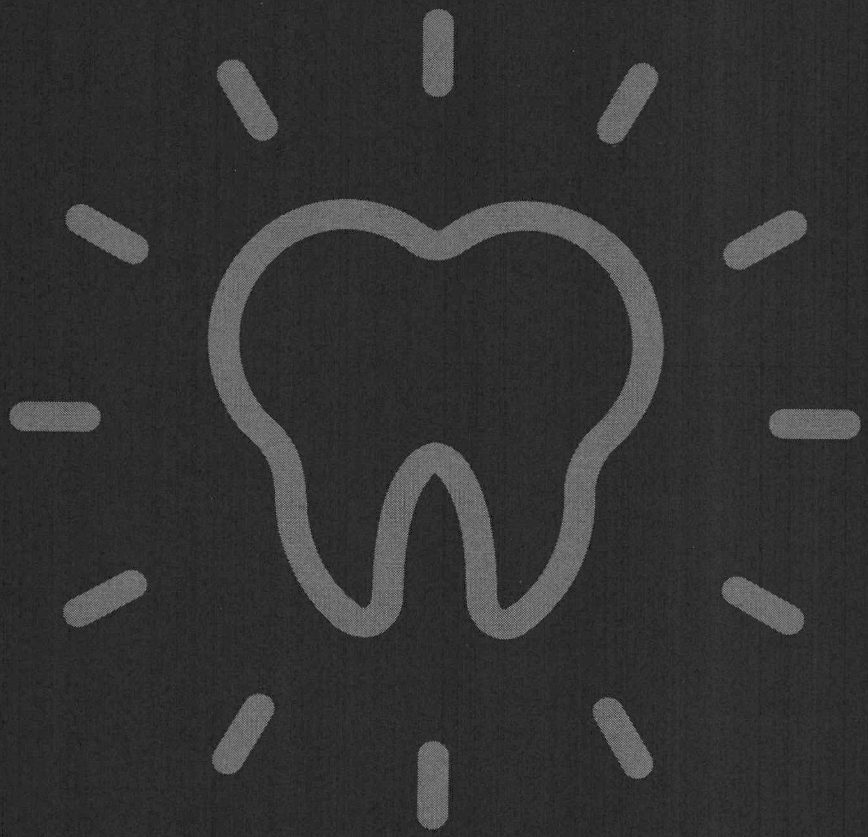

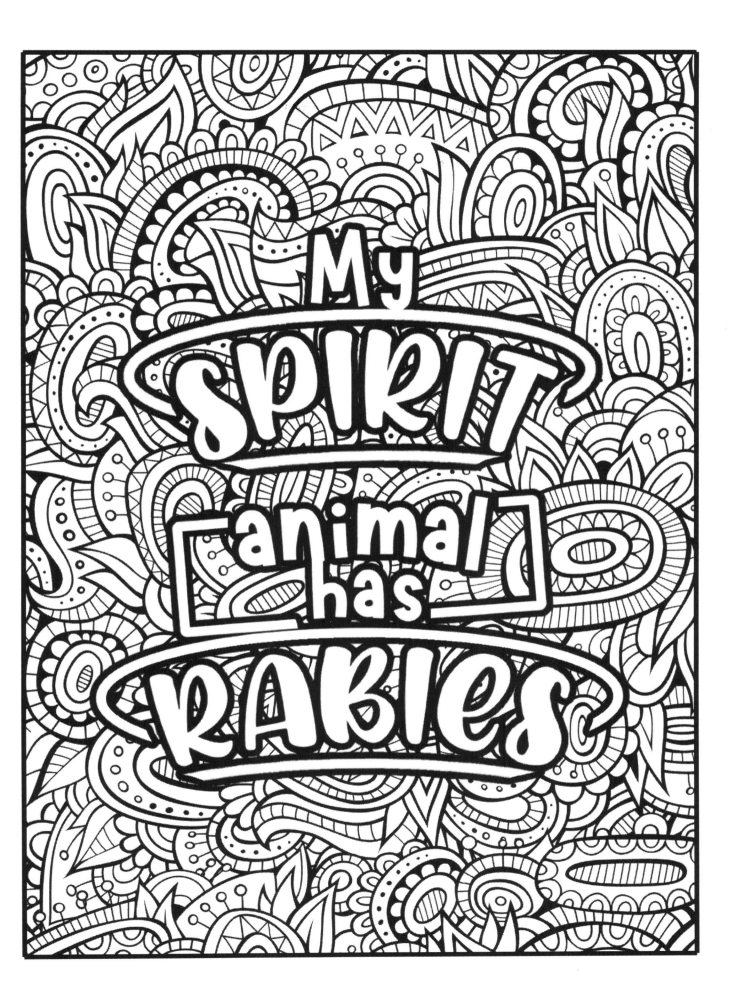

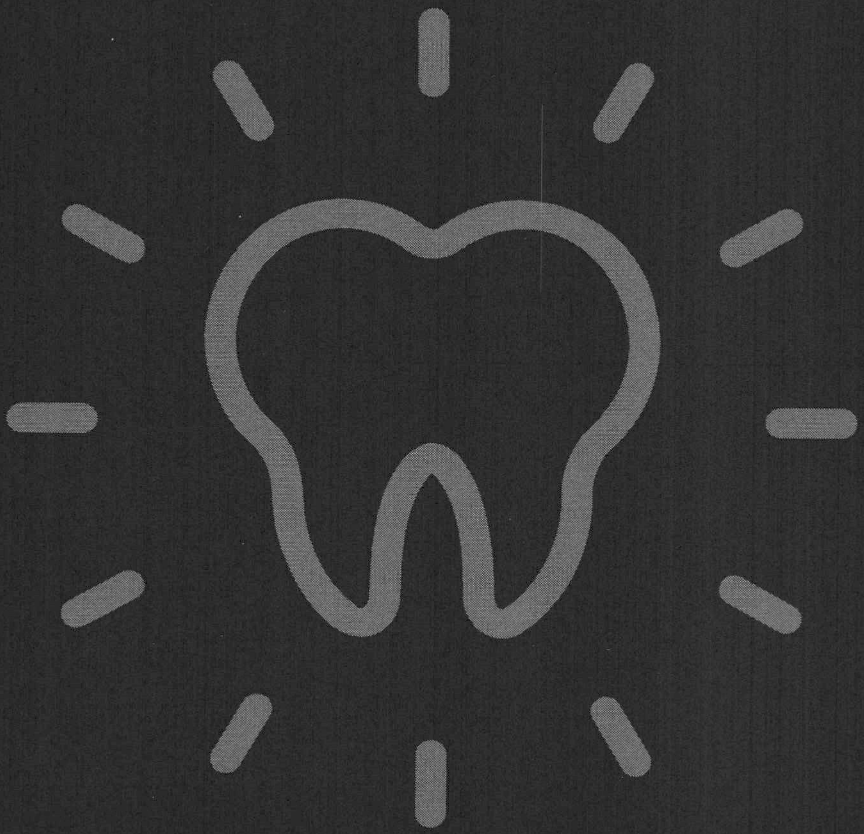

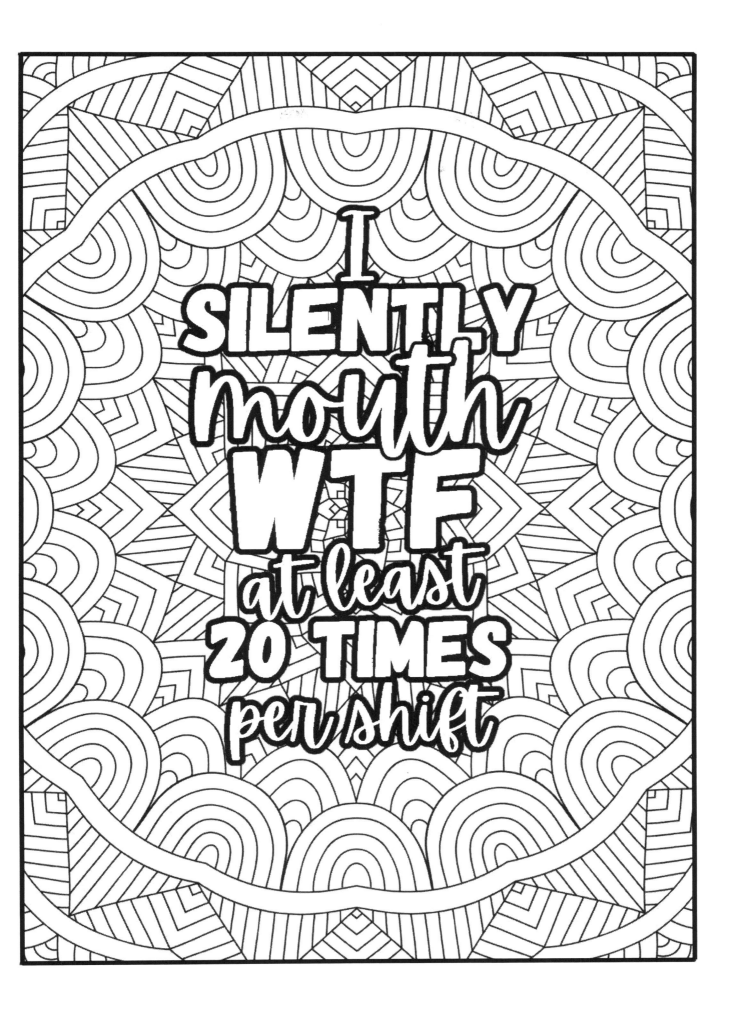

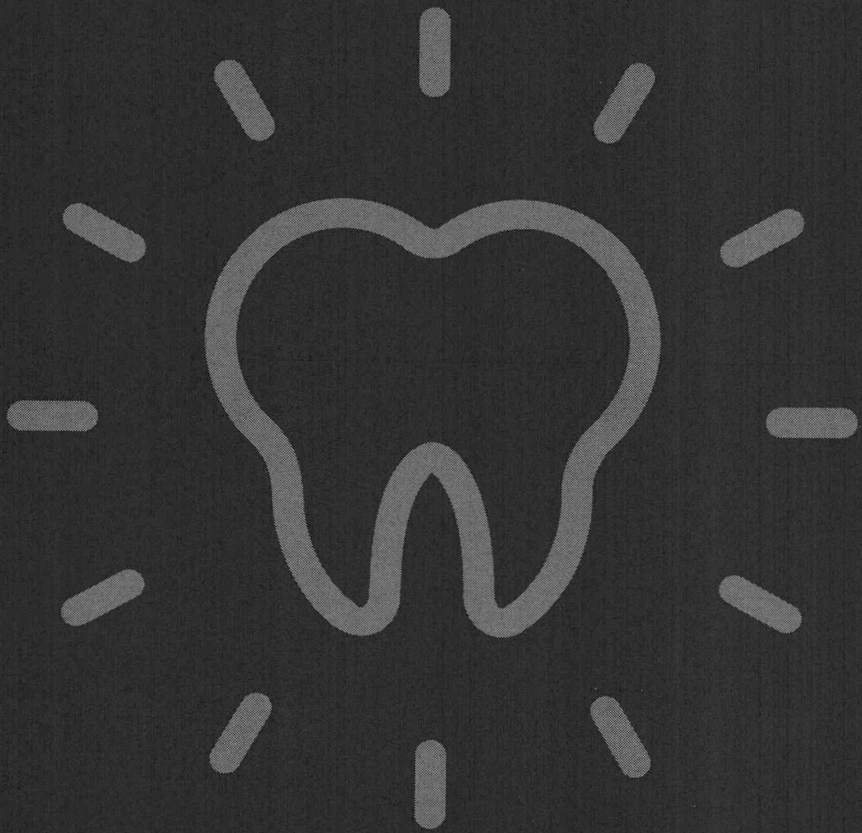

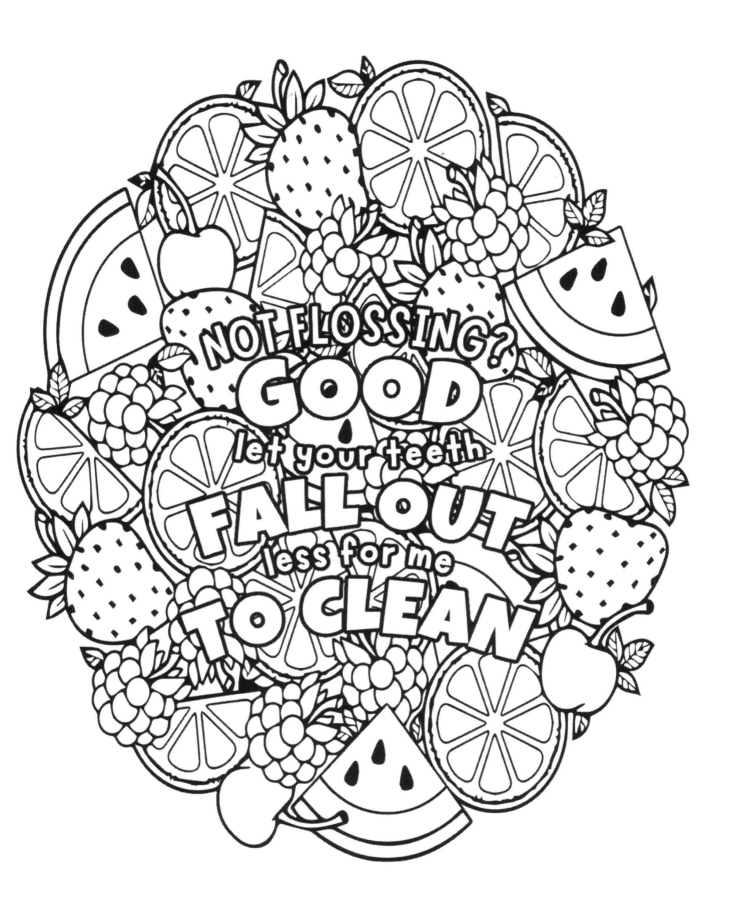

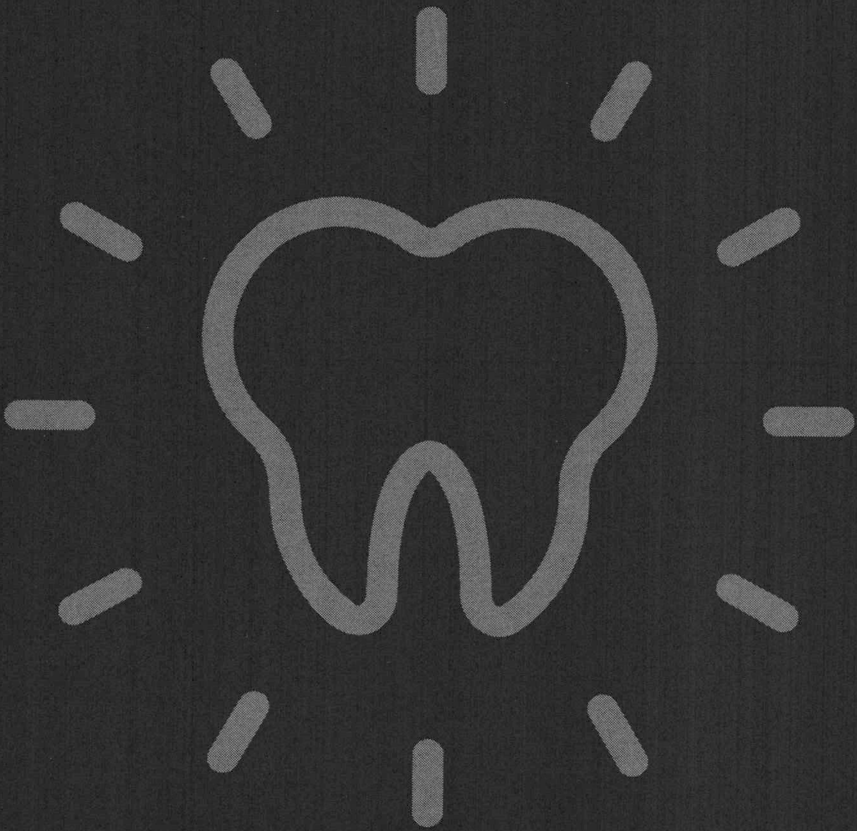

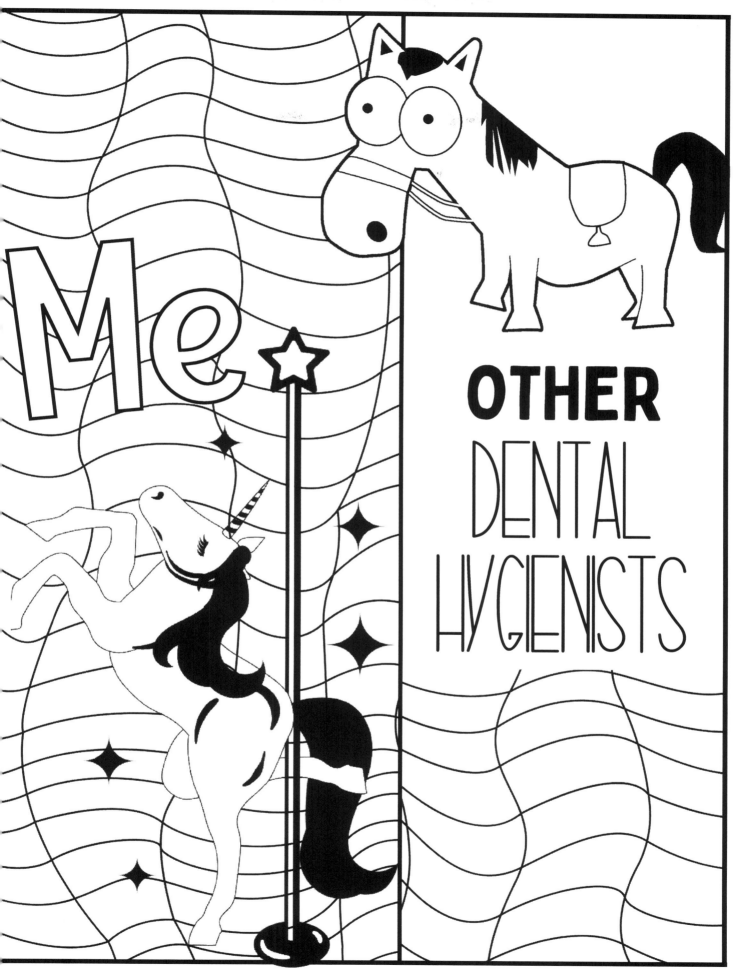

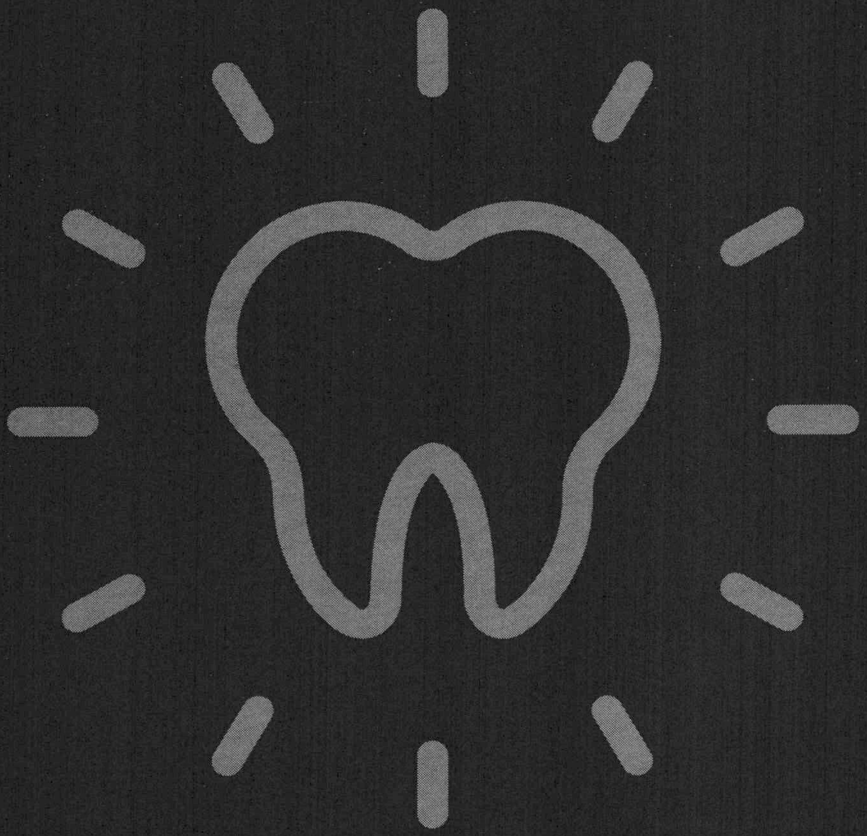

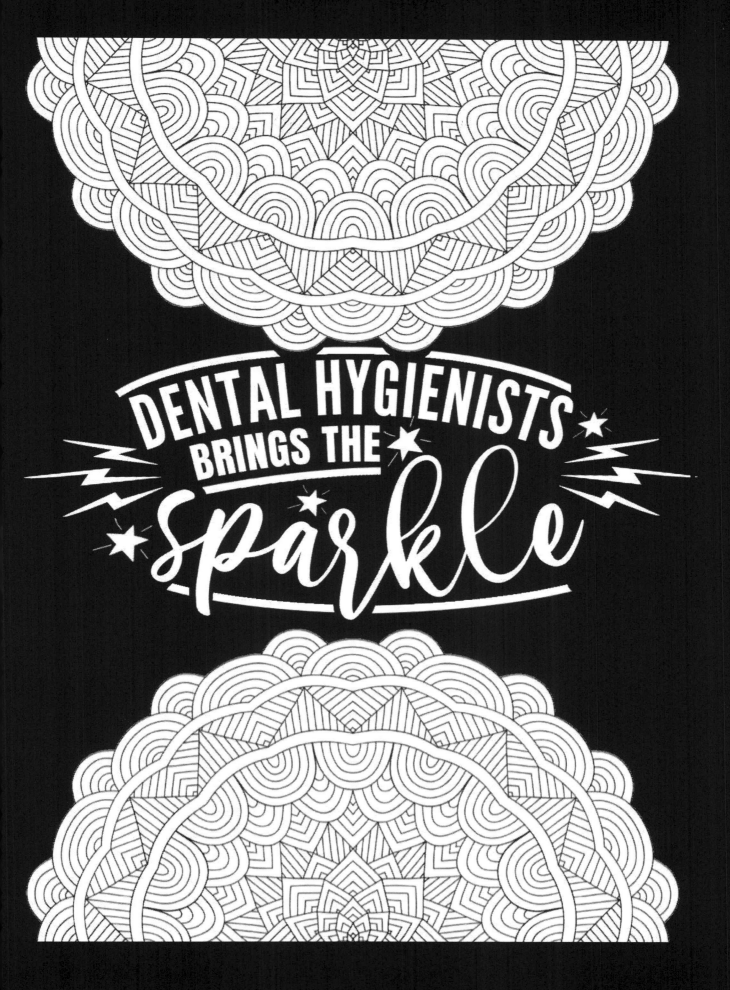

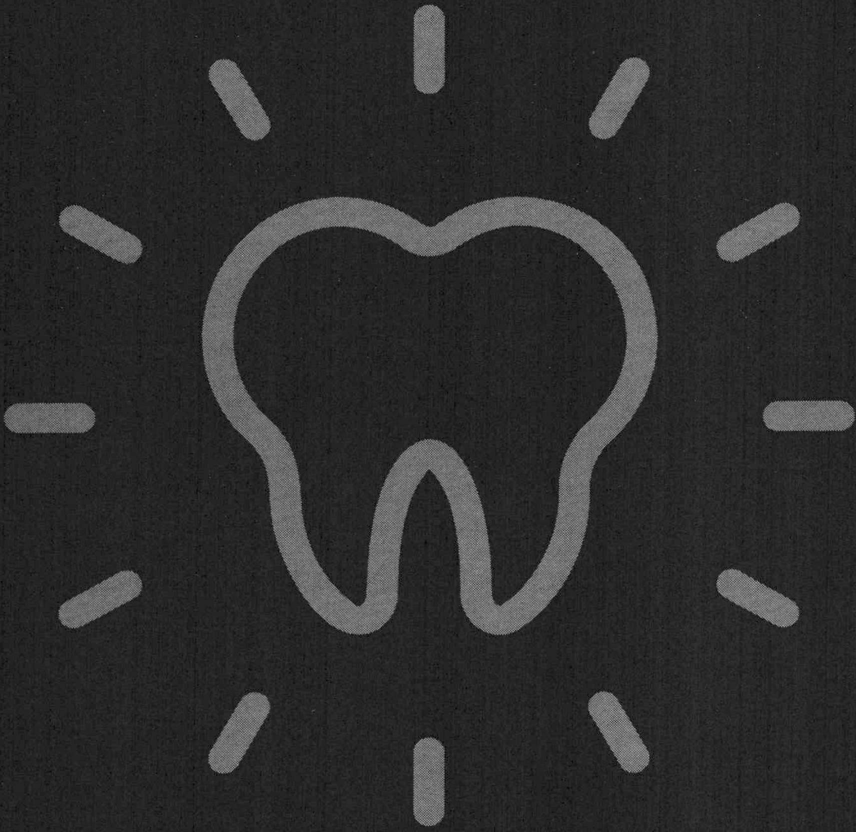

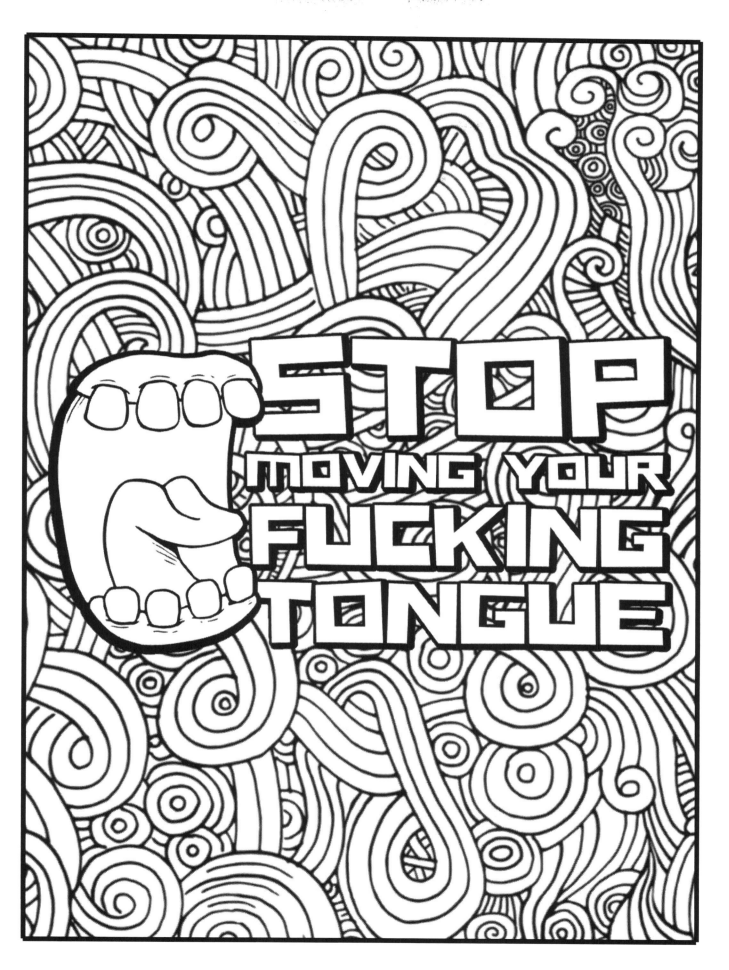

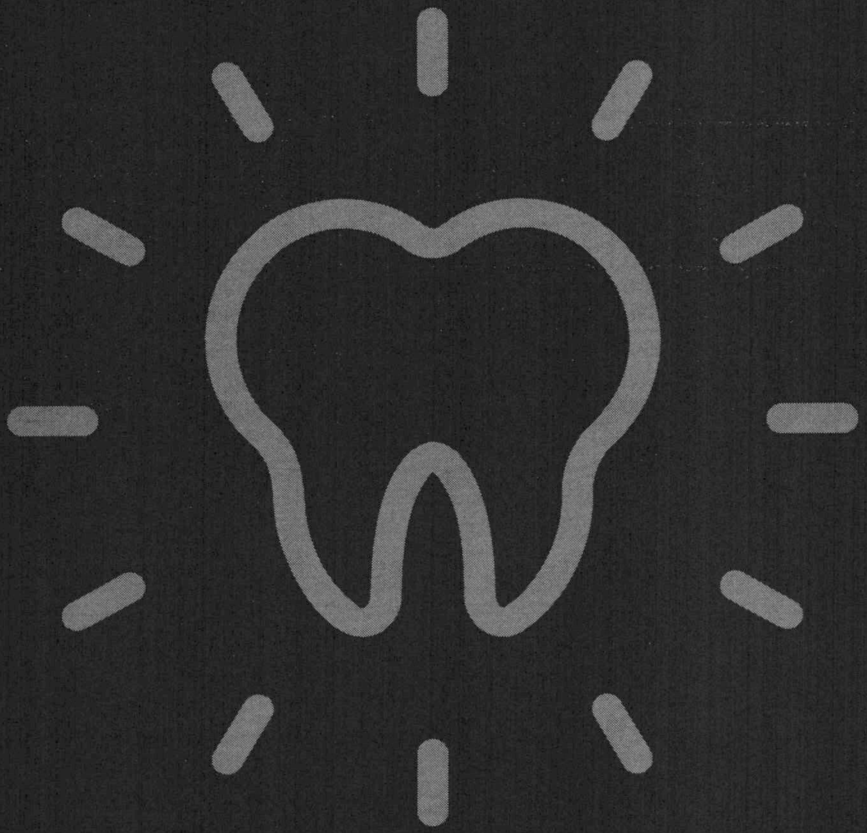

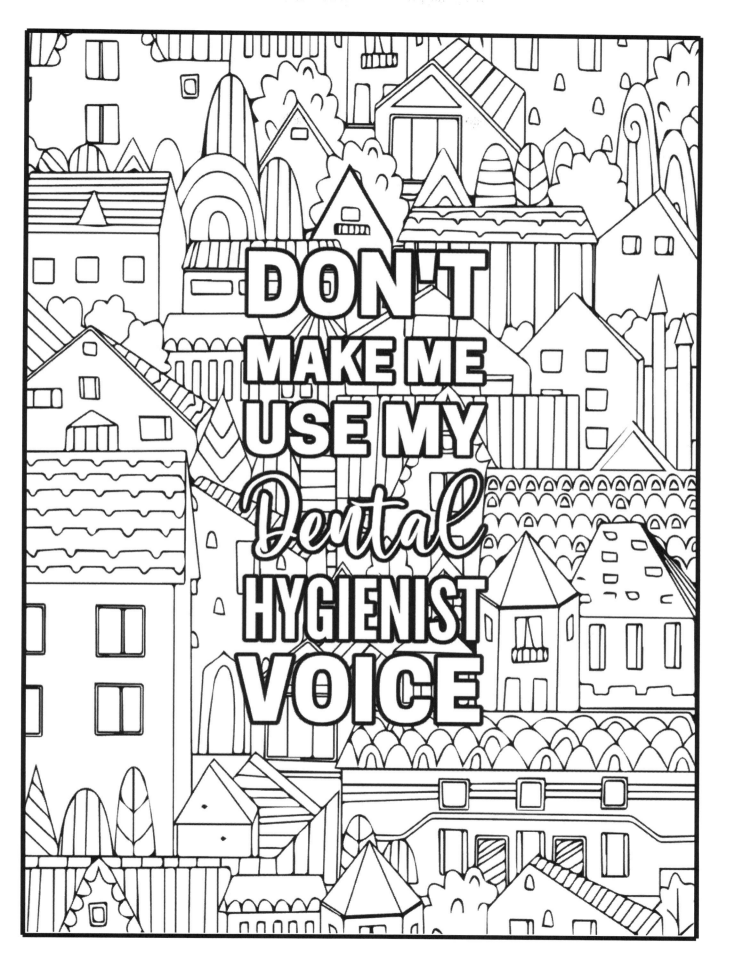

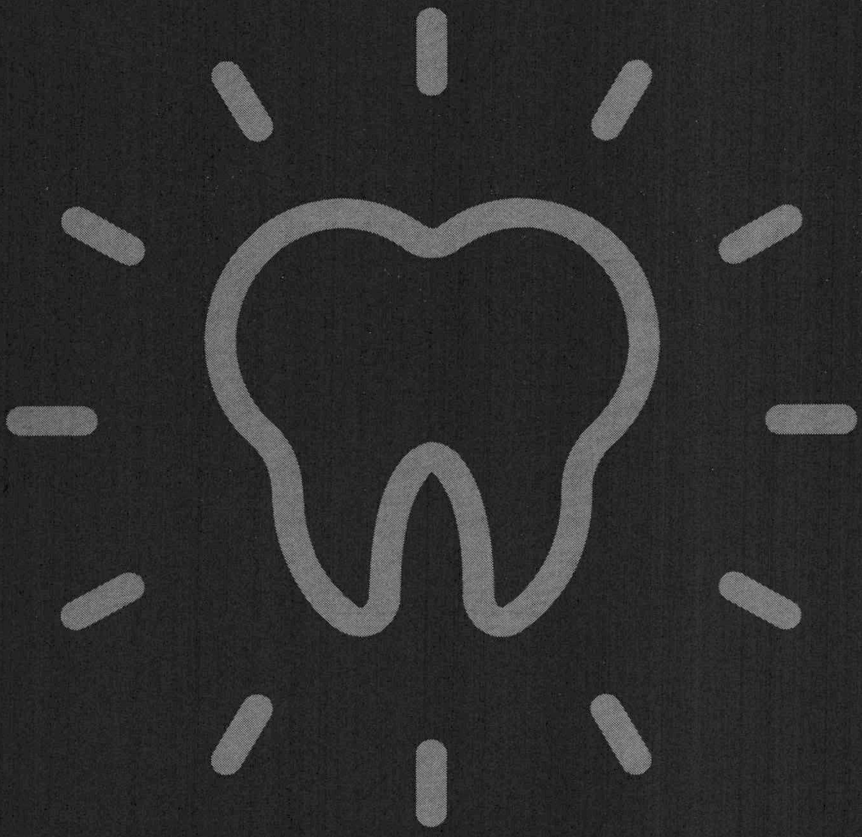

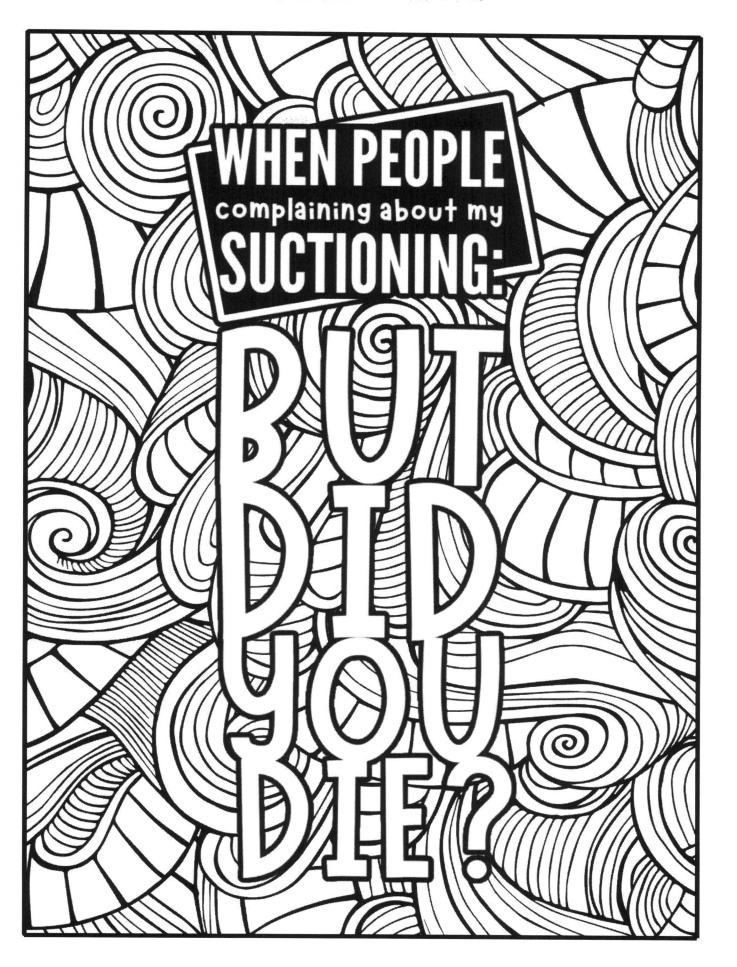

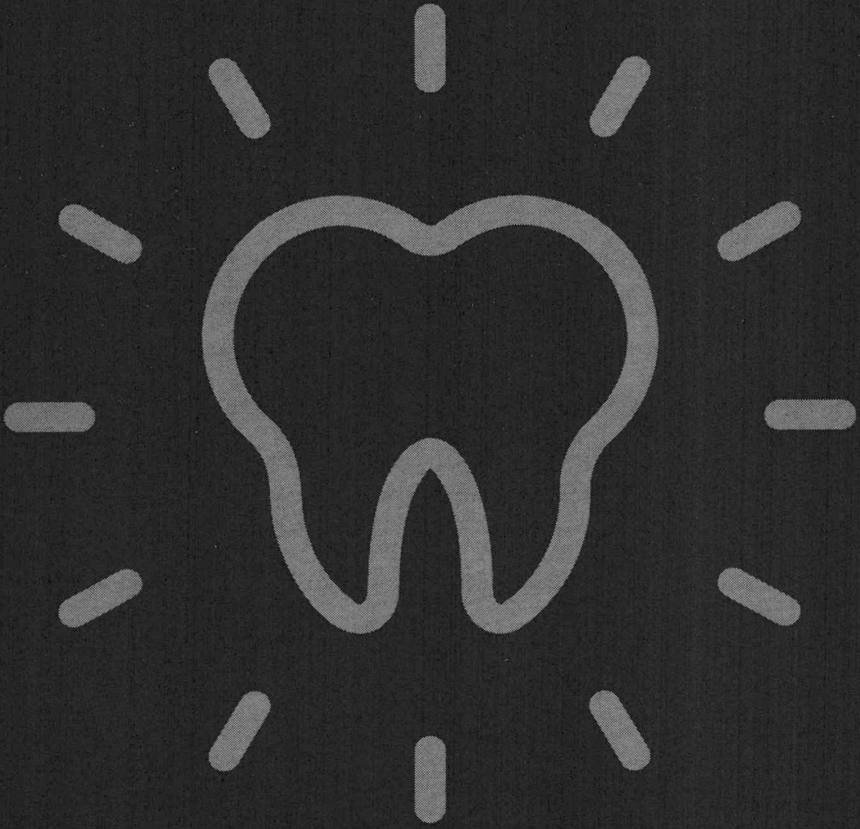

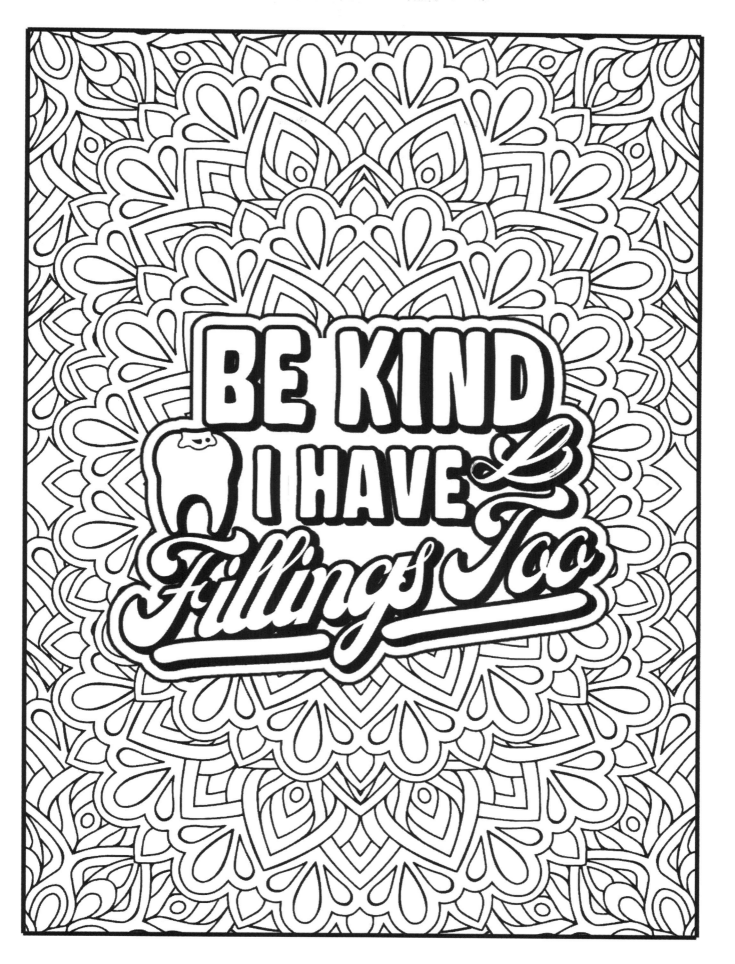

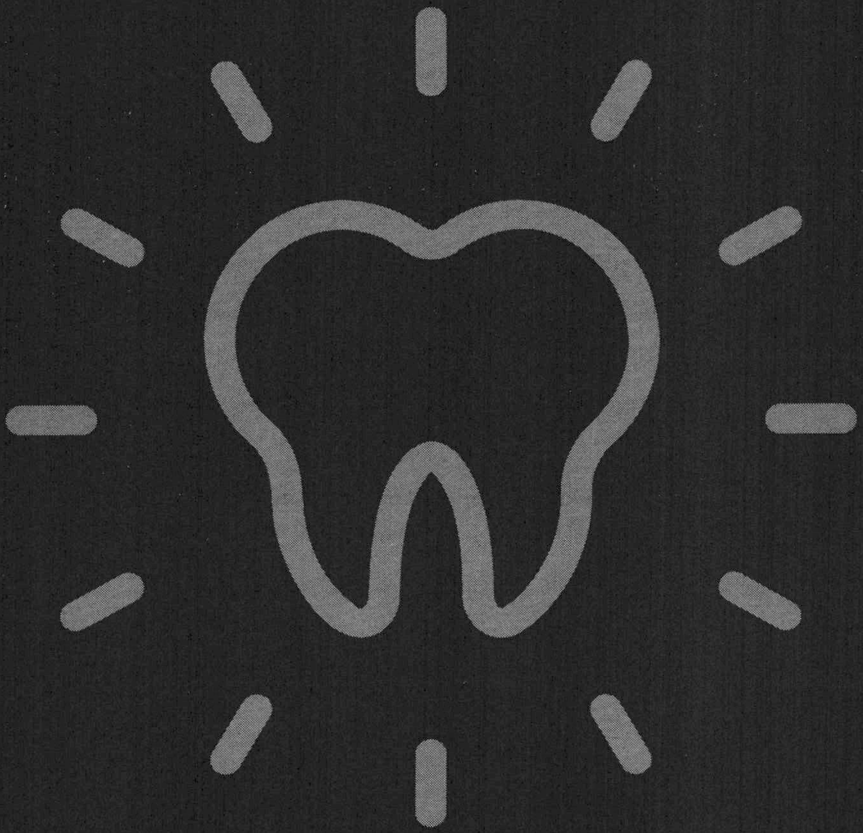

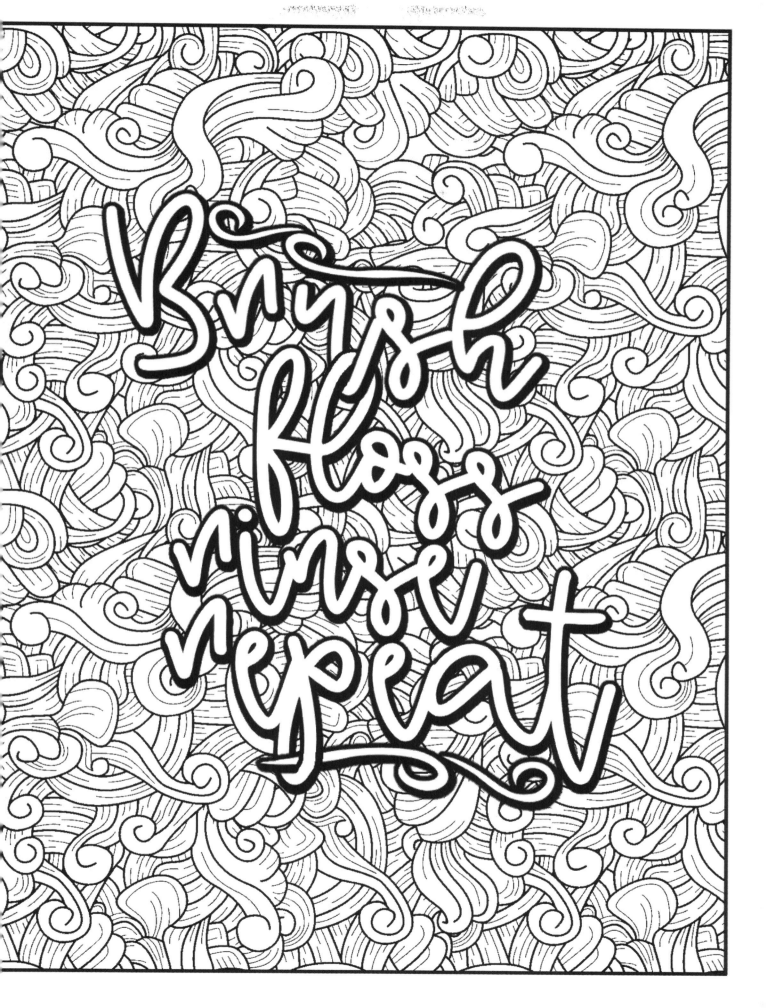

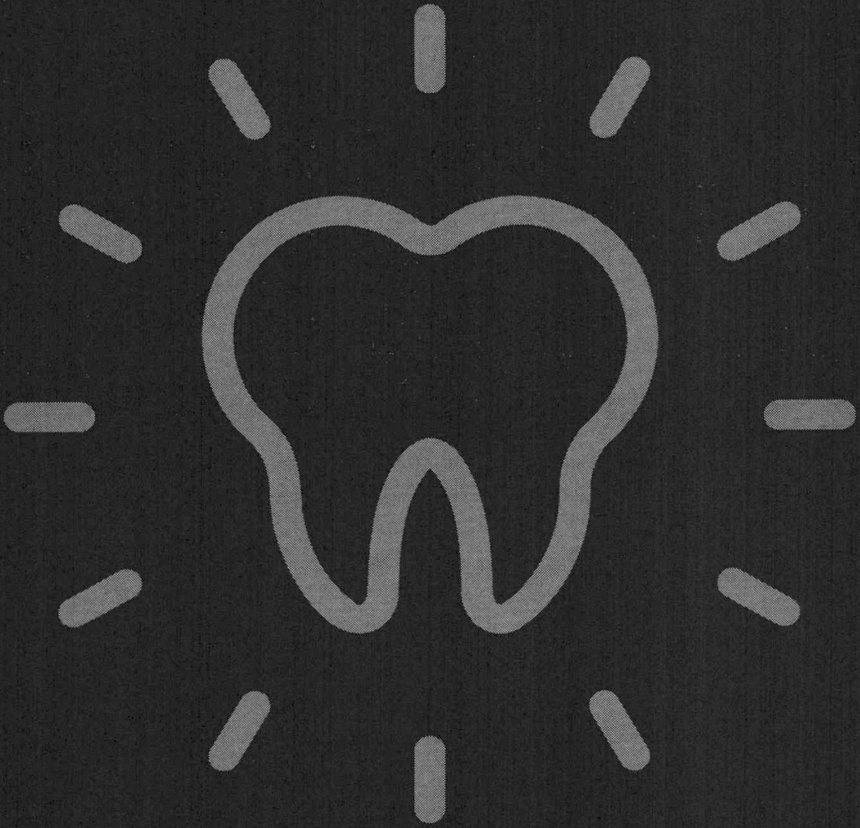

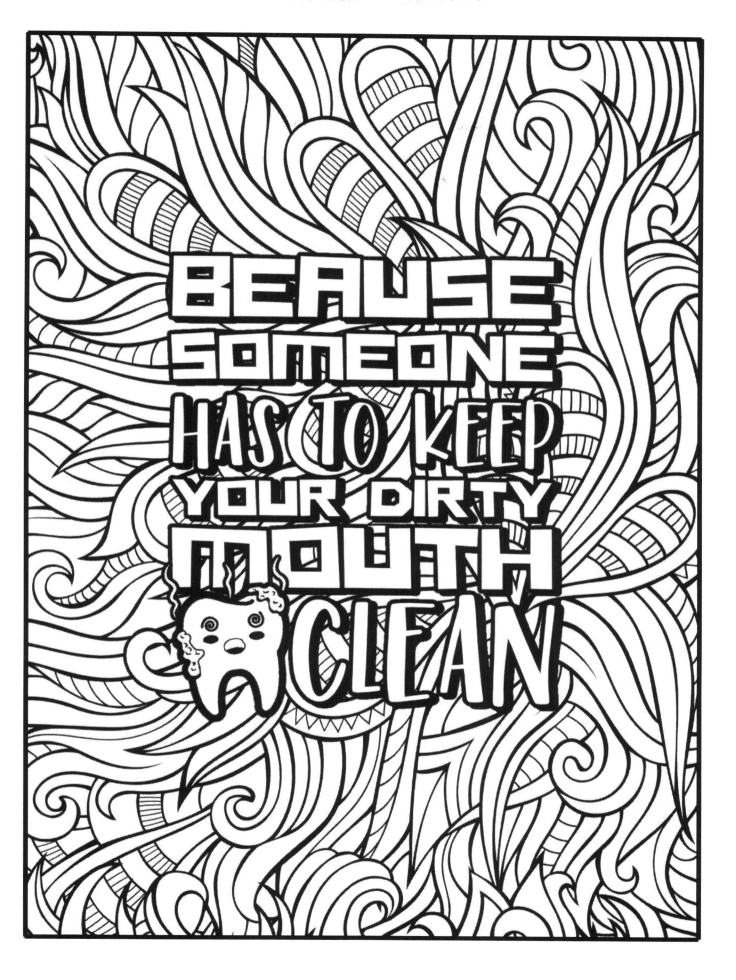

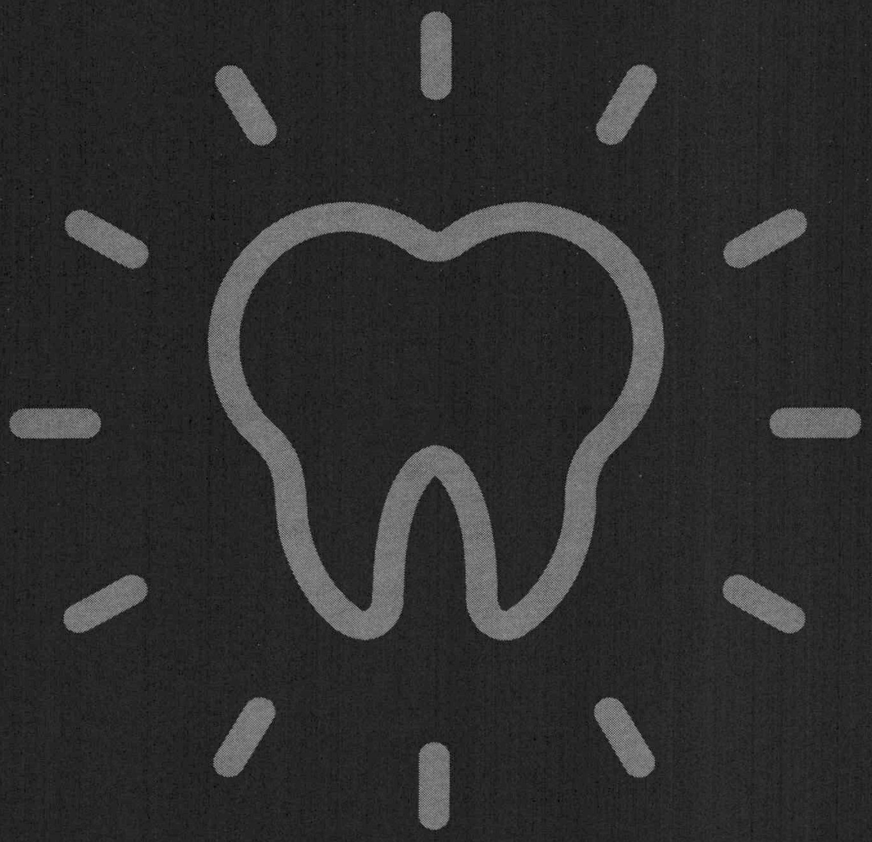

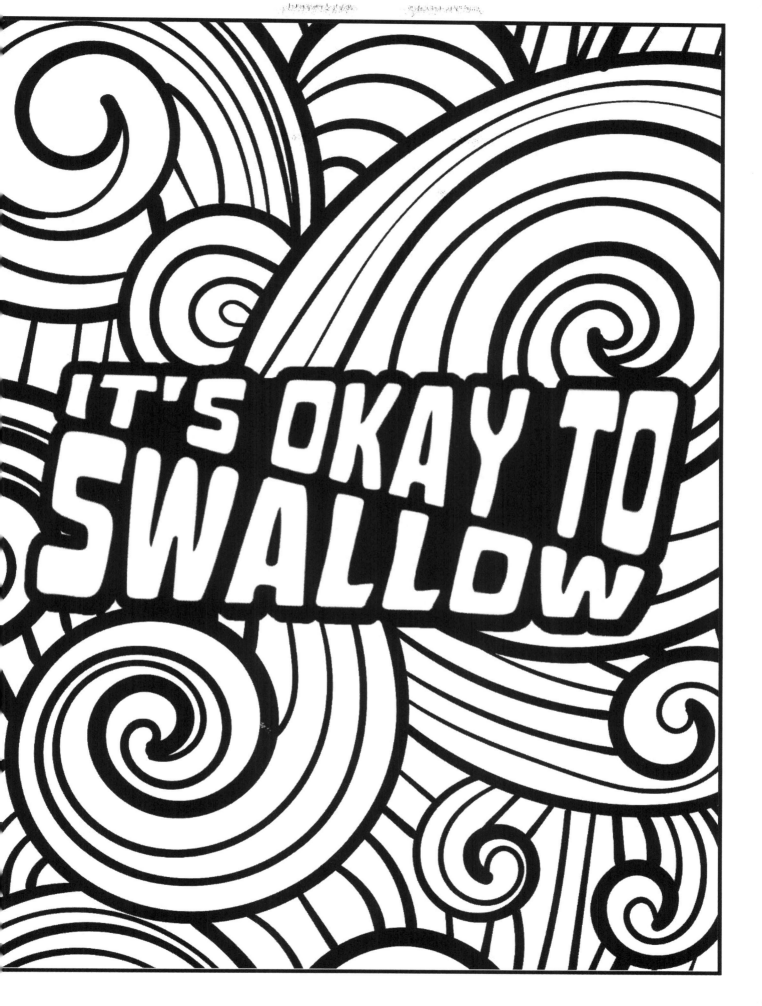

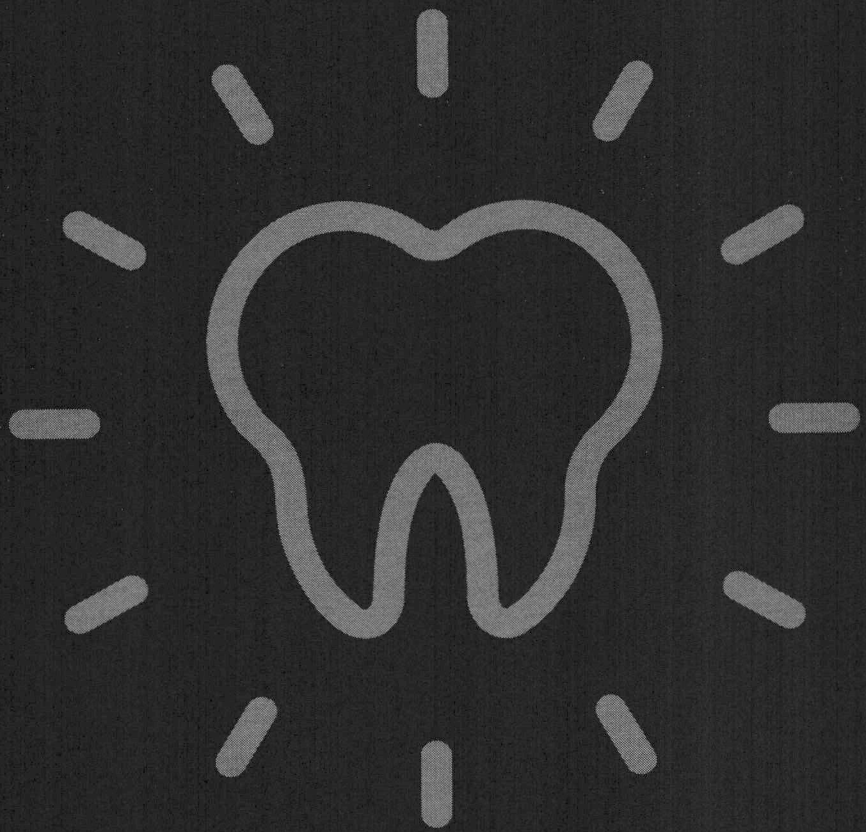

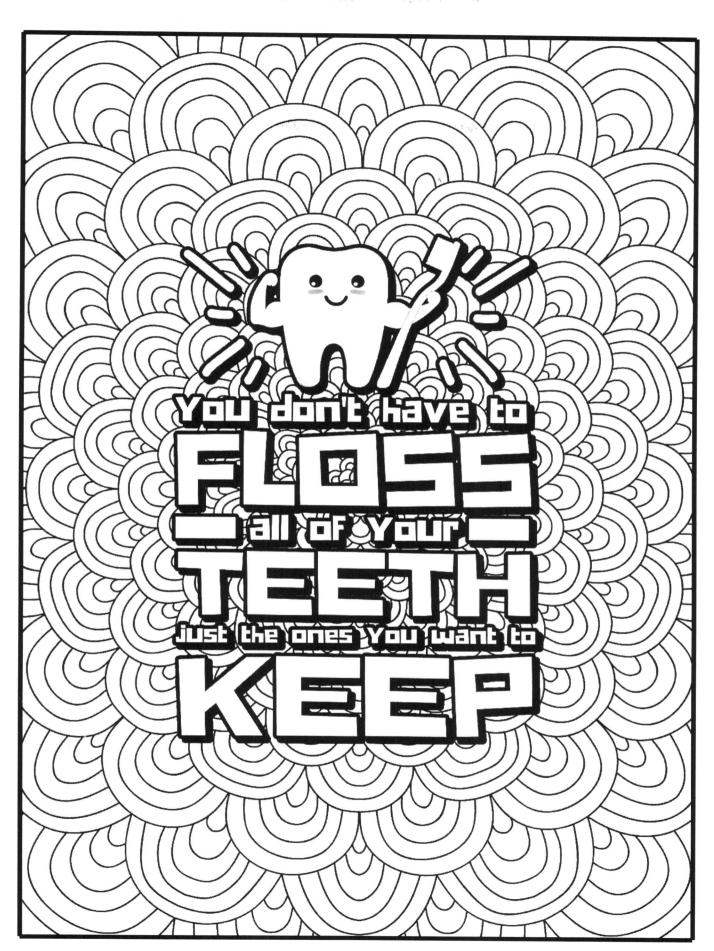

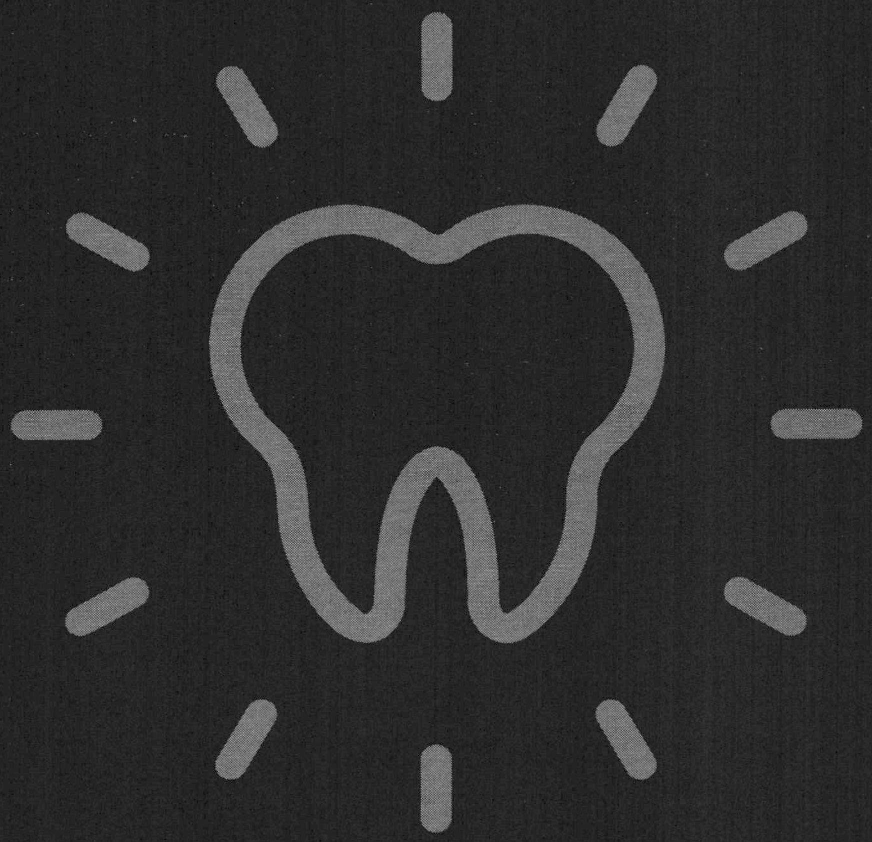

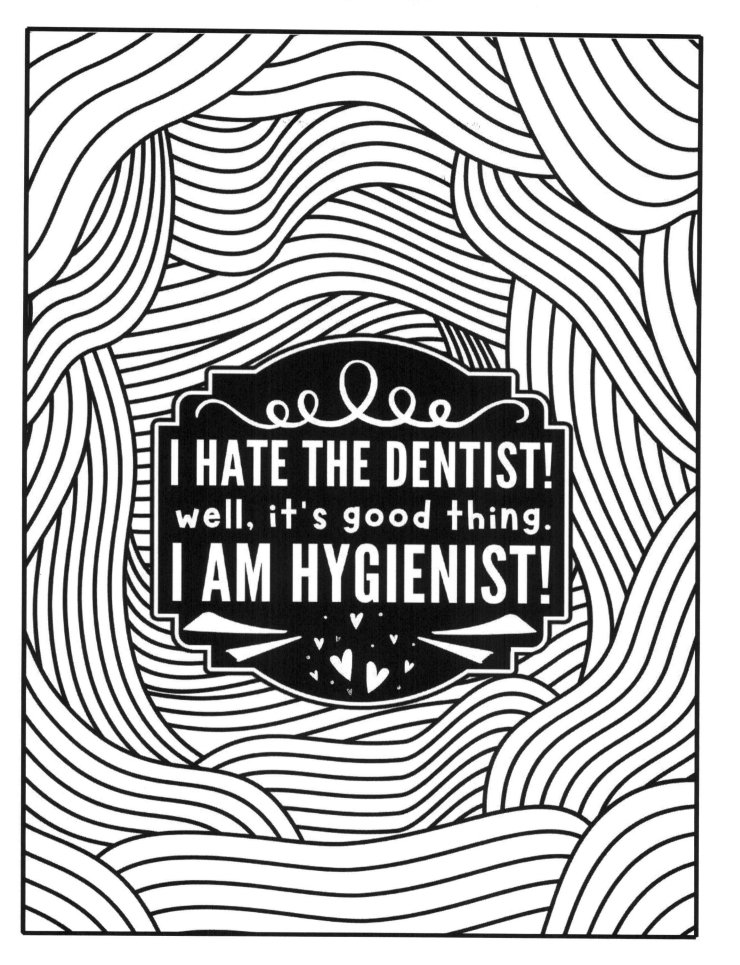

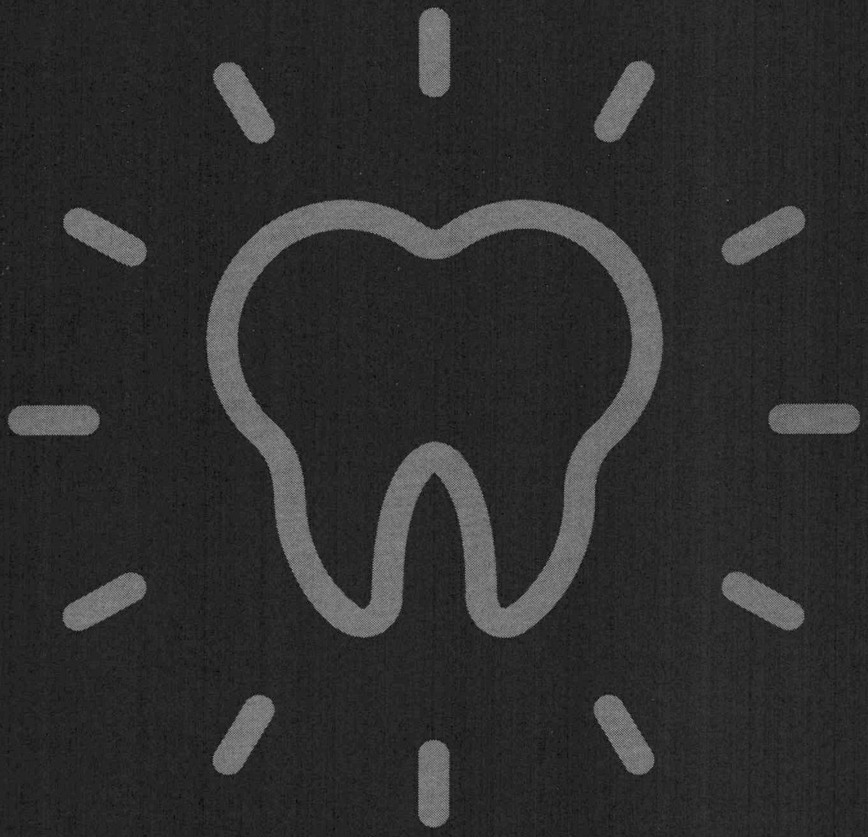

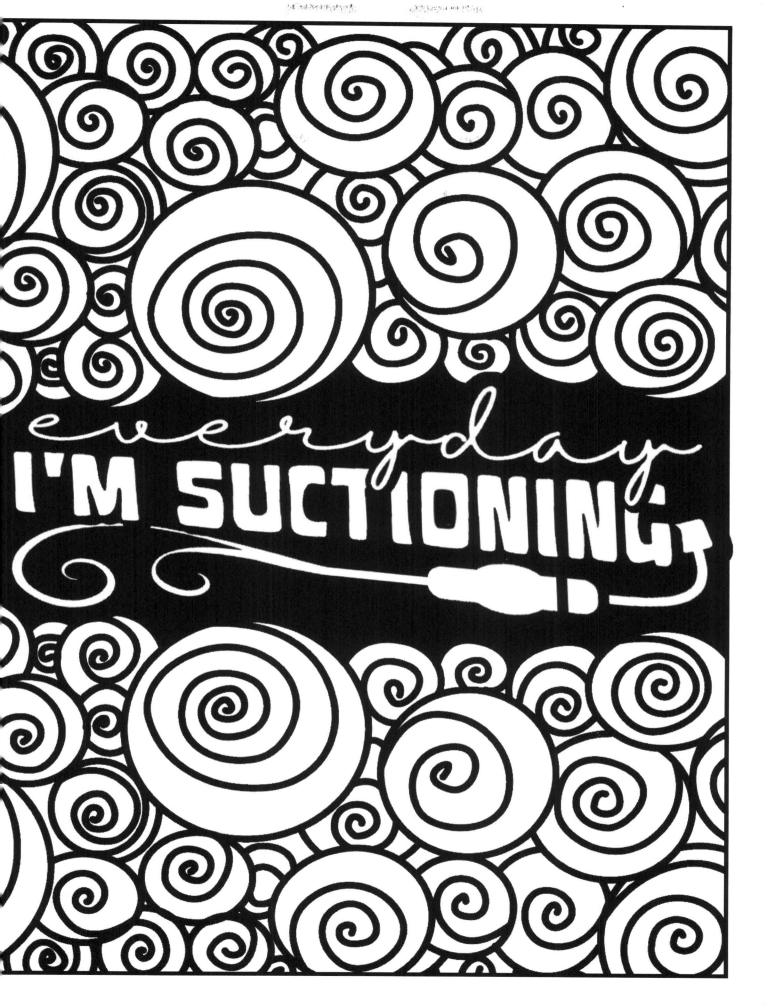

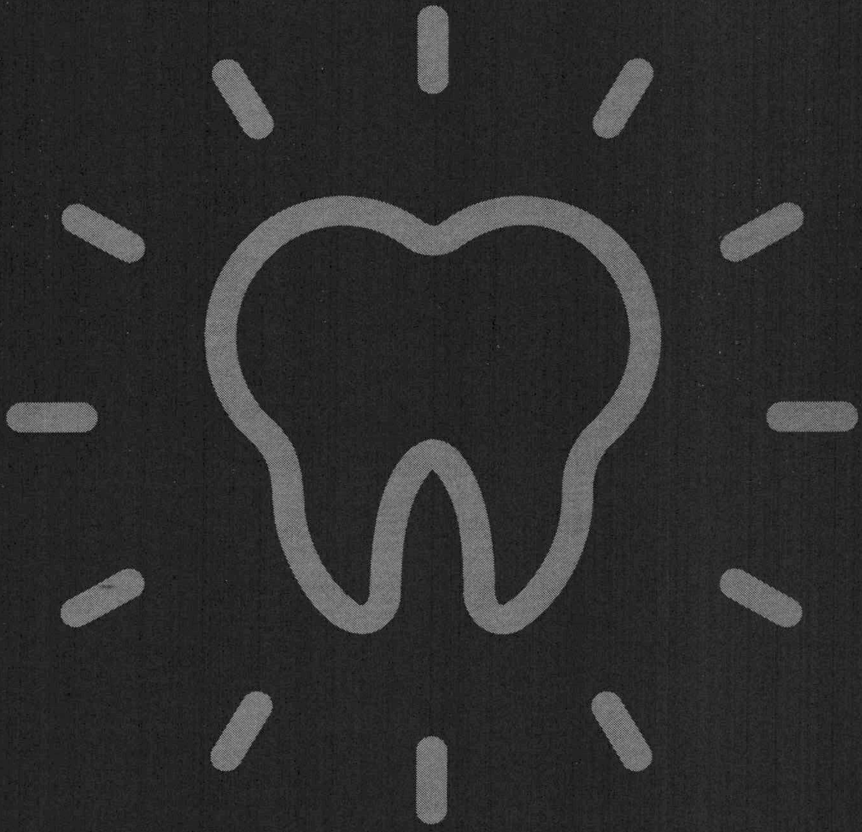

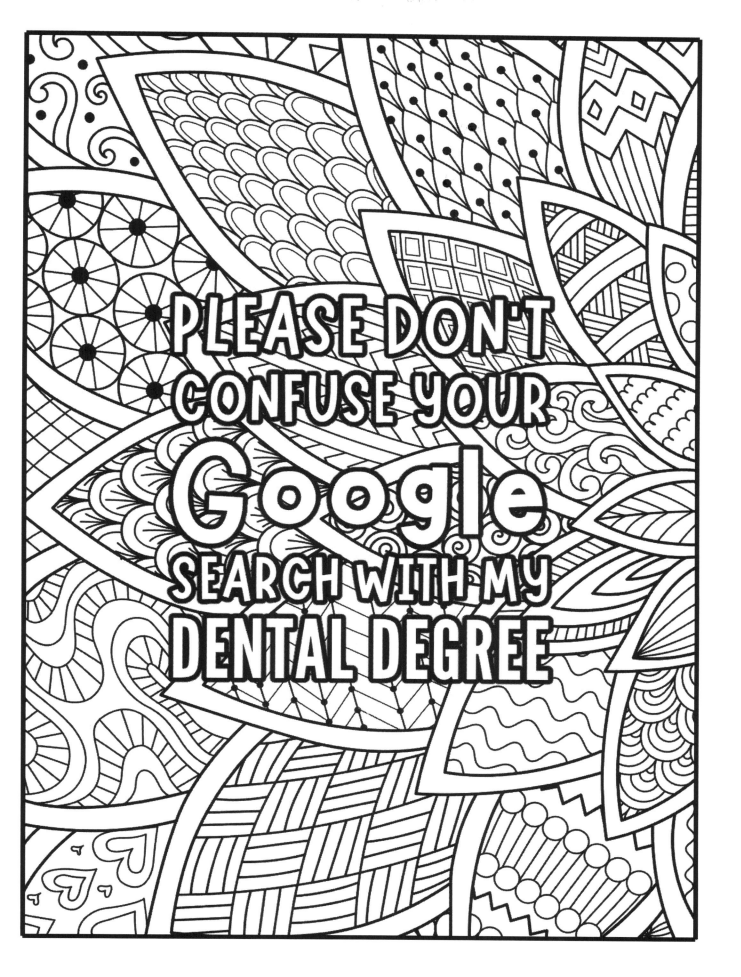

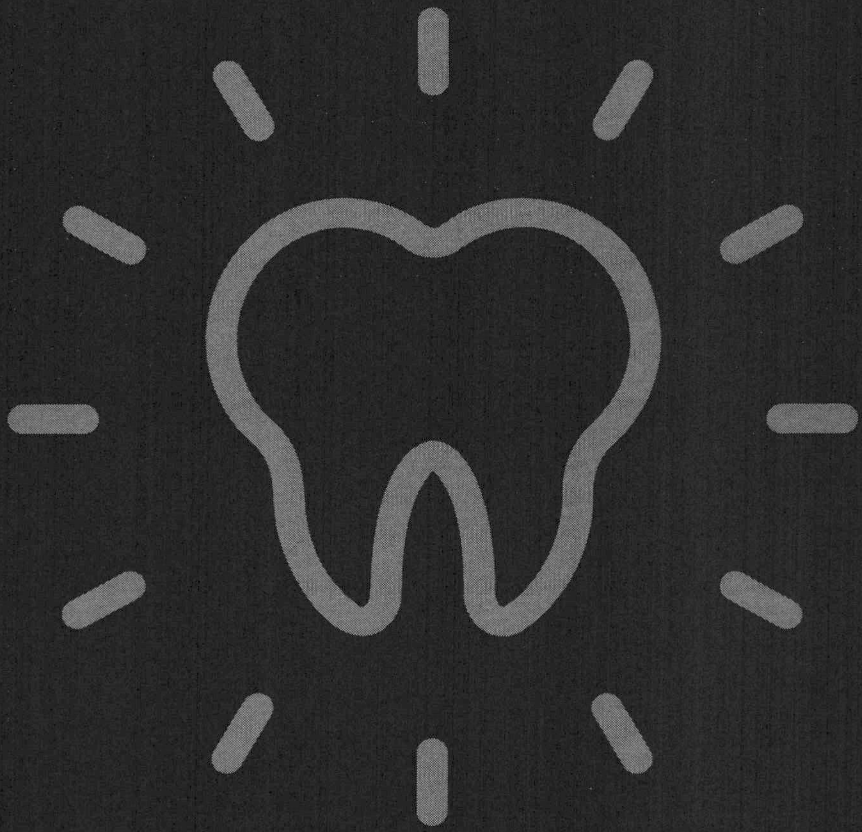

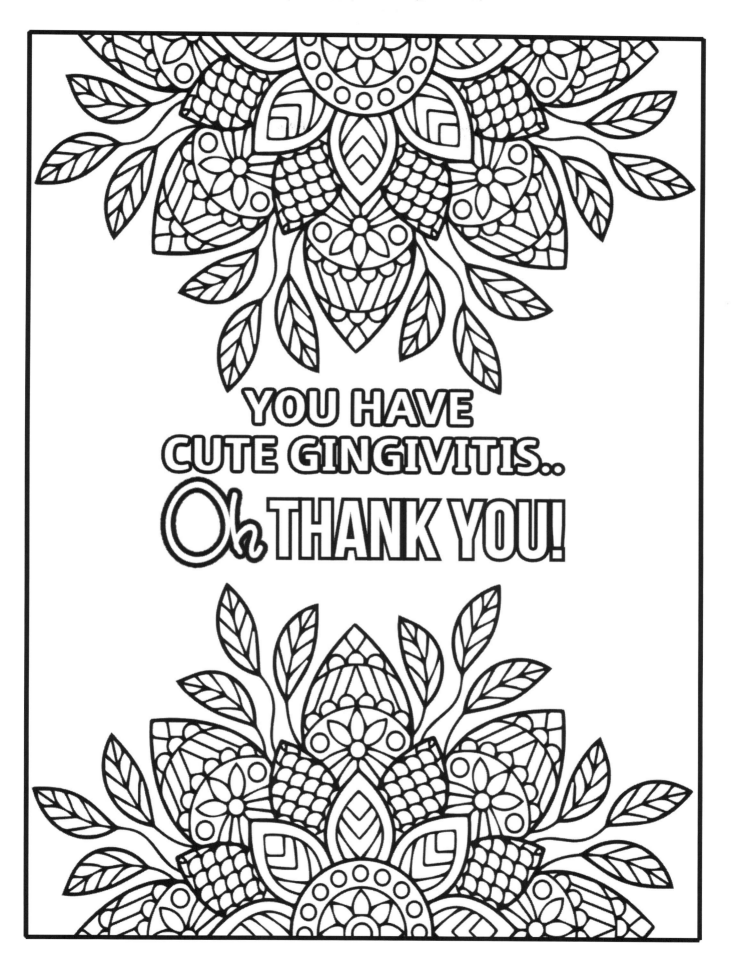

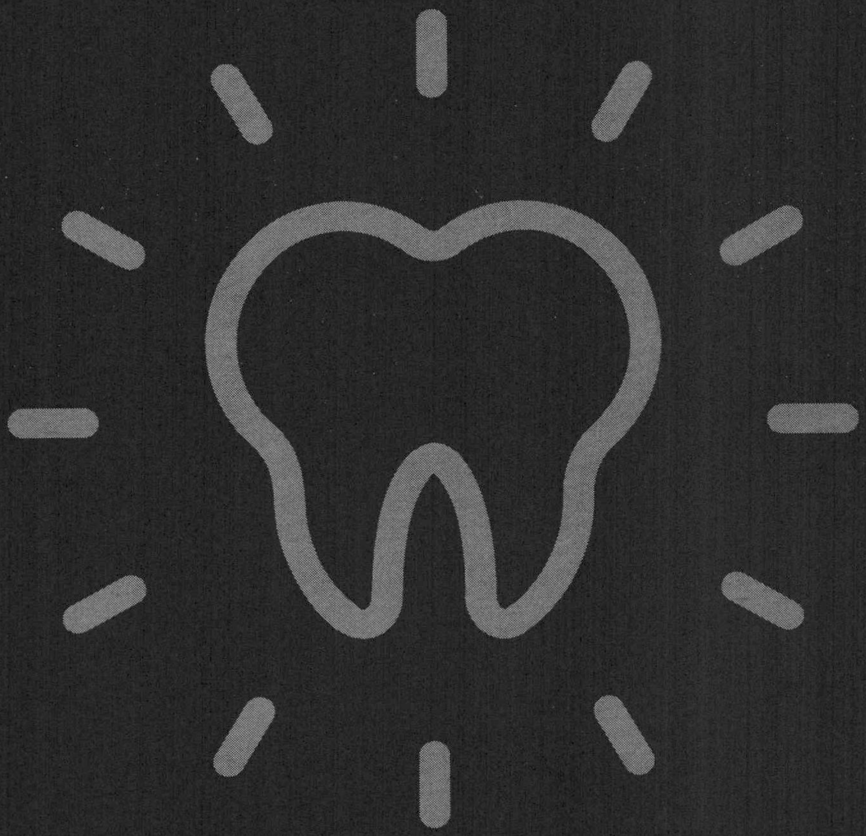

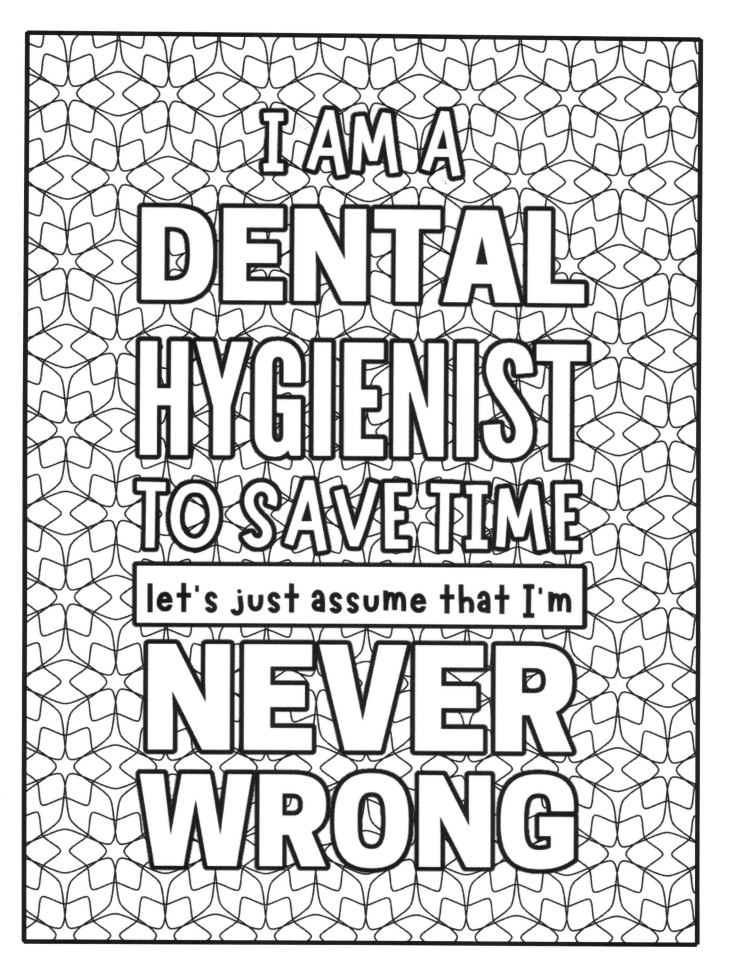

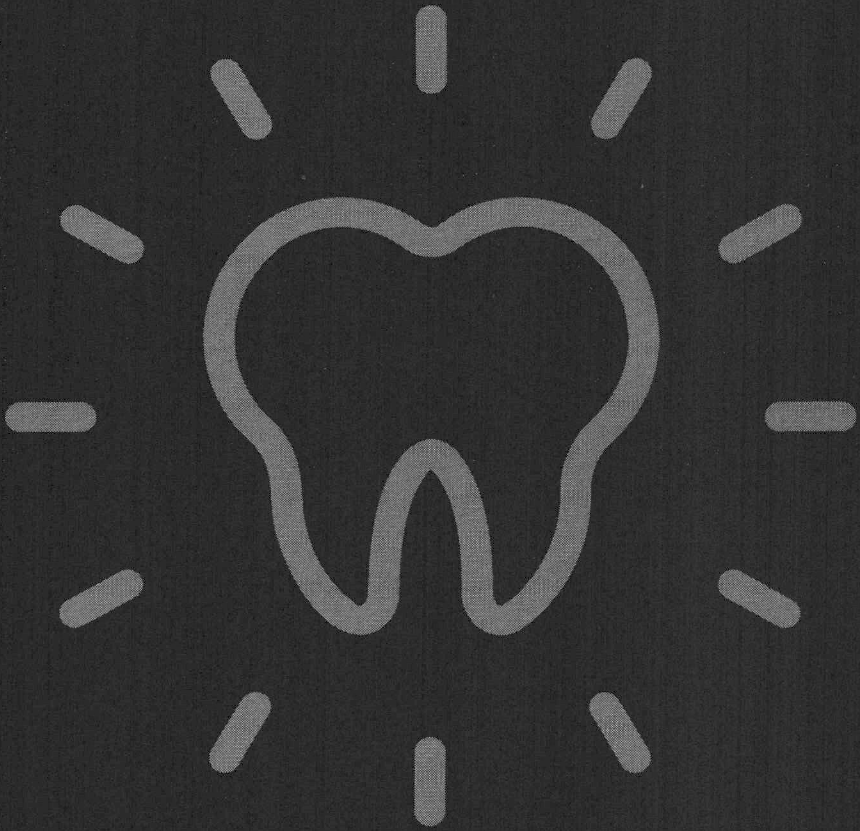

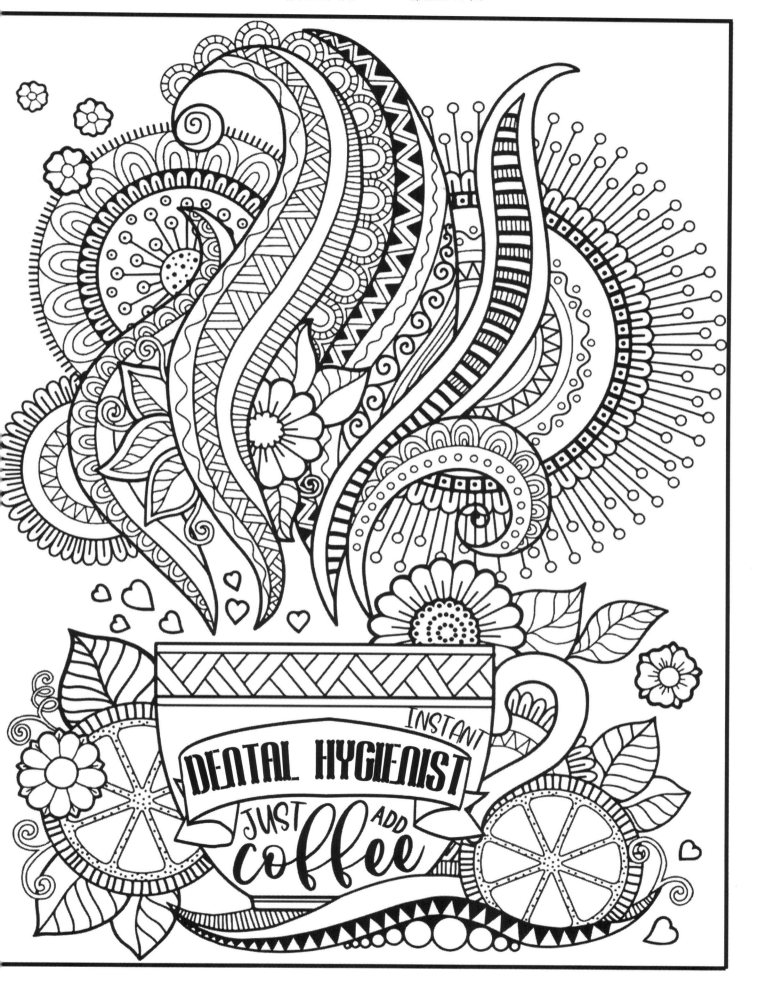

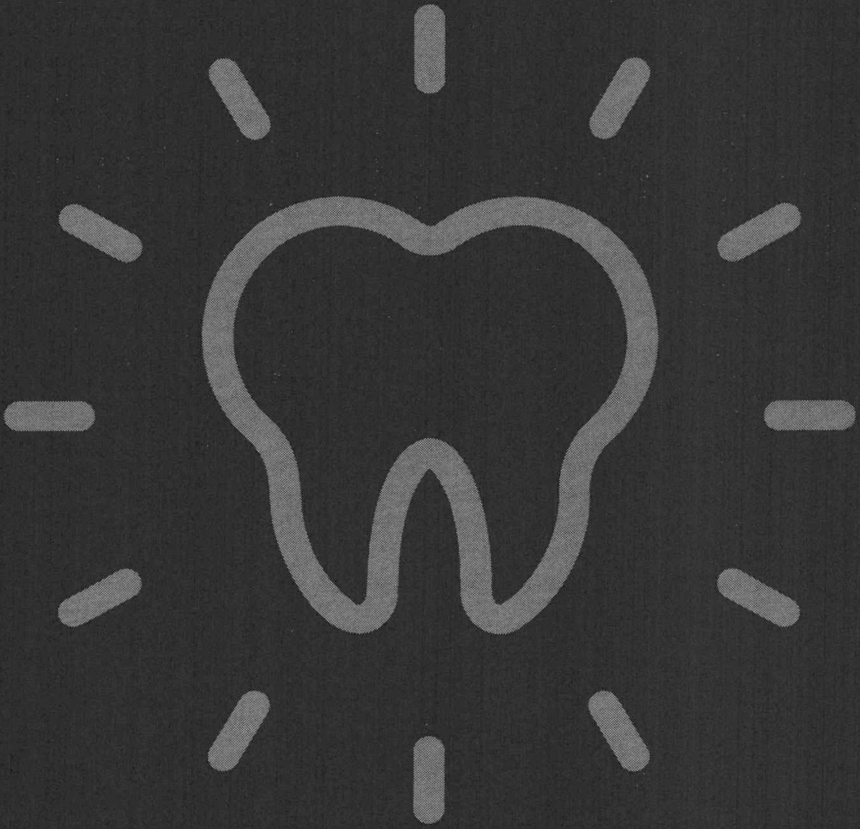

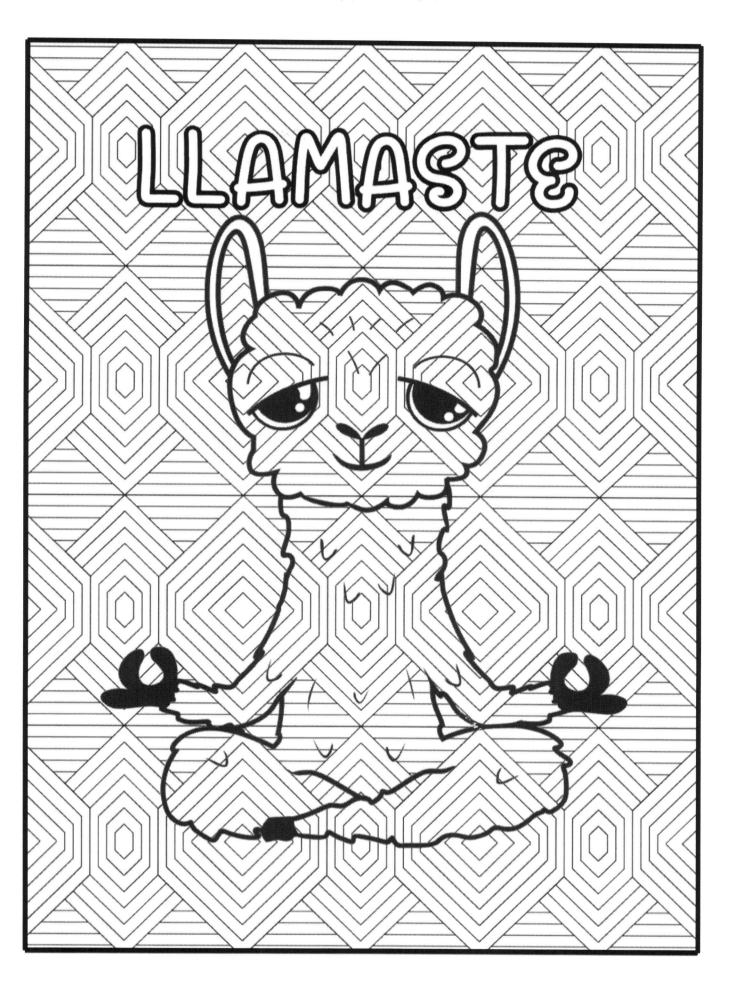

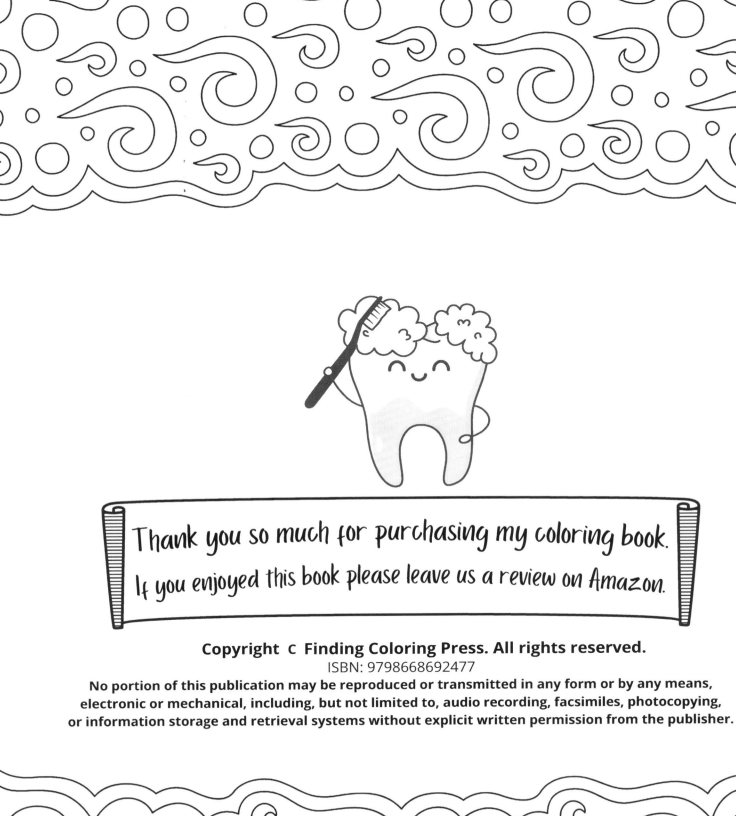

Thank you so much for purchasing my coloring book.

If you enjoyed this book please leave us a review on Amazon.

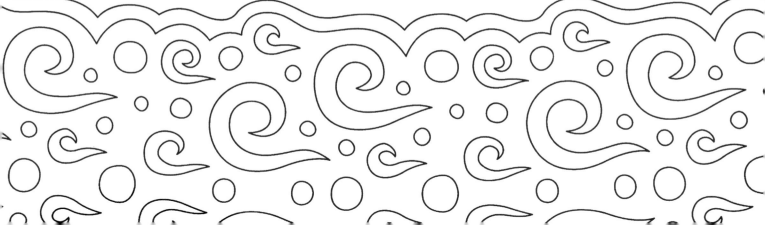

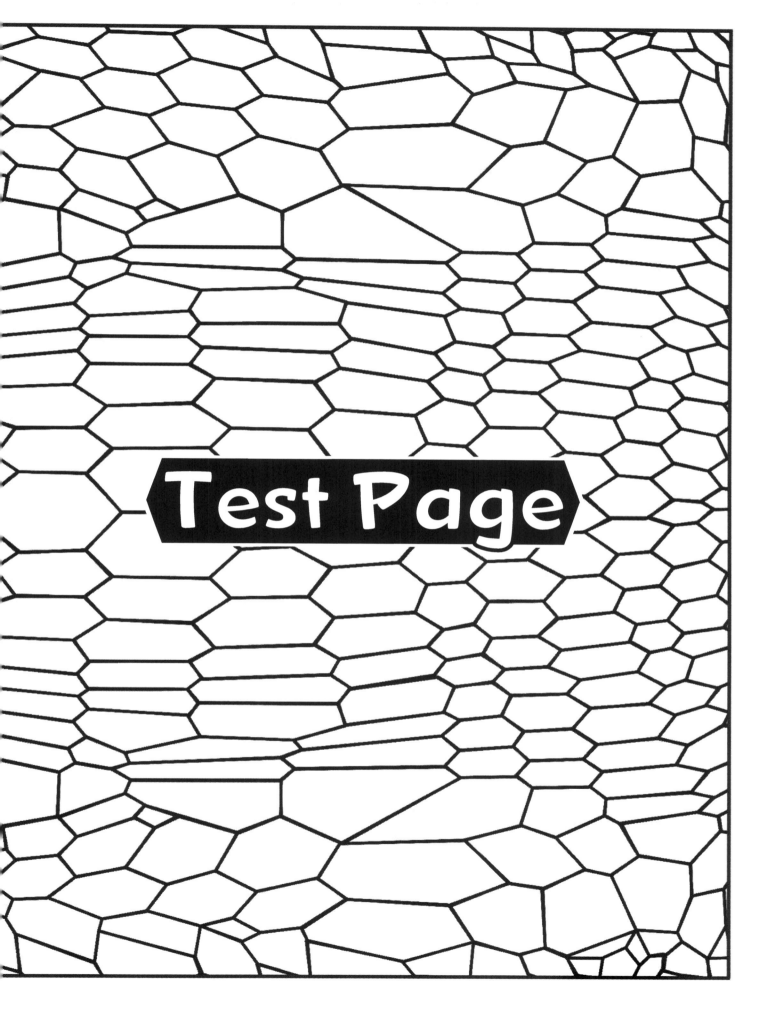

Printed in Great Britain
by Amazon